BIOMECHANICS OF BODY MOVEMENT IN SPORTS

Vijay Lakshmi

KHEL SAHITYA KENDRA
7/26, Ansari Road, Daryaganj,
New Delhi-110002

Published by:
KHEL SAHITYA KENDRA
7/26, Ansari Road, Darya Ganj, New Delhi-110002
Ph.: (O) 011-65190343, 43551324, 42564726
(M) 9811088729, (Fax) 011-42564726
(Res.) 47091605
E-mail: khelsahitya1@rediffmail.com
Web: www.khelsahitya.com, www.kskpublisher.com

ISBN 978-81-7524-316-3

PRINTED IN INDIA 2026

Printed by:
ASIAN OFFSET PRINTERS
Delhi

Laser Typesetting by:
JAIN MEDIA GRAPHICS
Delhi

Preface

Through the years its meaning of Biomechanics has been extended to cover the study of the motions of all kinds of particles and continua, including quanta, atoms, molecules, gases, liquids, solids, structures, stars, and galaxies. In a generalized sense it is applied to the analysis of any dynamic system. Thus thermodynamics, heat and mass transfer, cybernetics, computing methods, etc., are considered proper provinces of mechanics. The biological world is part of the physical world around us and naturally is an object of inquiry in mechanics. Biomechanics seeks to understand the mechanics of living systems. Biomechanics is the study of the action of forces in promoting movement or equilibrium. It is important to many engineering disciplines.

To enjoy all that life has to offer, humans rely on the proper function and movement of muscles, bones, joints and other connective tissues. These tissues all work together to generate, absorb, redirect and manage physical forces.

Biomechanics of Body Movements in Sports

Chapter 1

Introduction to Biomechanics

History of Biomechanics

The Study of Locomotion

Instruction concerning a dislocation of a vertebra of the neck: if you examine a man having a dislocation of the a vertebra of his neck, should you find him unconscious of his arms and legs on account of it, then you should say an ailment which cannot be treated

The seventeen columns on the recto comprise the first surgical treatise thus far discovered. It consists exclusively of case reports, systematically organized - beginning with injuries of the head and proceeding downward through the body, like a modern treatise on anatomy. The treatment of these injuries is rational and chiefly surgical; there is resort to magic in only one case out of the forty-eight cases preserved. Each case is classified by one of three different verdicts: (1) favorable, (2) uncertain, or (3) unfavorable. The third verdict, expressed in the words, 'an ailment not to be treated,' is found in no other Egyptian medical treatise. This unfavorable verdict occurring fourteen times in the Edwin Smith Papyrus marks a group of cases (besides one more case) which the surgeon cannot cure. It is likely that the patients described in the 48 cases were injured by falls (maybe from working on monuments or buildings) or were victims of battle (many wounds appear to be caused by spears, clubs or daggers.) The brain is mentioned 7 times throughout the papyrus. However, there is no use of the word "nerve."

The 48 cases contained within Edwin Smith Surgical Papyrus concern:

- 27 head injuries
- 6 throat and neck injuries
- 2 injuries to the clavicle (collarbone)
- 3 injuries to the arm
- 8 injuries to the sternum (breastbone) and ribs
- 1 injury to the shoulder
- 1 injury to the spine

Edwin Smith, was born in Connecticut in 1822, the year that Egyptian hieroglyphic was first deciphered. On January 20, 1862 in the city of Luxor, Smith bought the surgical papyrus from a dealer named Mustapha Aga. Two months later the same vandals sold him the remaining fragments glued onto a dummy roll. Although Smith recognized the fraud, pieced the two together, and made an attempt at translation, it was not until 1930 that James H. Breasted translated the treatise and established its importance. According to Breasted, the Edwin Smith Papyrus is a copy of an ancient composite manuscript which contained, in addition to the original author's text (3000-2500 B.C.), a commentary added a few hundred years later in the form of 69 explanatory notes (glosses). It contains 48 systematically arranged case histories, beginning with injuries of the head and proceeding downward to the thorax and spine, where the document unfortunately breaks off. These cases are typical rather than individual, and each presentation of a case is divided into title, examination, diagnosis, and treatment.

The scribe of over 3,500 years ago had copied at least eighteen columns of the venerable treatise and had reached the bottom of a column when, pausing in the middle of a line, in the middle of a sentence, in the middle of a word, he laid down his pen and pushed aside forever the great Surgical Treatise he had been copying, leaving 15½ inches (39 cm.) bare and unwritten at the end of his roll.

Case Eight

Title: Instructions concerning a smash in his skull under the skin of his head.

Examination: If thou examinest a man having a smash of his skull, under the skin of his head, while there is nothing at all upon it, thou shouldst palpate his wound. Shouldst thou find that there is a swelling protruding on the out side of that smash which is in his skull, while his eye is askew because of it, on the side of him having that injury which is in his skull; (and) he walks shuffling with his sole, on the side of him having that injury which is in his skull..

Treatment: His treatment is sitting, until he [gains color], (and) until thou knowest he has reached the decisive point.... Gloss: As for: "He walks shuffling with his sole," he (the surgeon) is speaking about his walking with his sole dragging, so that it is not easy for him to walk, when it (the sole) is feeble and turned over, while the tips of his toes are contracted to the ball of his sole, and they (the toes) walk fumbling the ground. He (the surgeon) says: "He shuffles," concerning it.

Case Thirty-One

Title: Instructions concerning a dislocation in a vertebra of [his] neck. Examination: If thou examinest a man having a dislocation in a vertebra of his neck, shouldst thou find him unconscious of his two arms (and) his two legs on account of it, while his phallus is erected on account of it, (and) urine drops from his member without his knowing it; his flesh has received wind; his two eyes are bloodshot; it is a dislocation of a vertebra of his neck extending to his backbone which causes him to be unconscious of his two arms (and) his two legs. If, however, the middle vertebra of his neck is dislocated, it is an emissio seminis which befalls his phallus.

Diagnosis: Thou should stay concerning him: "One having a dislocation in a vertebra of his neck, while he is unconscious of his two legs and his two arms, and his urine dribbles. An ailment not to be treated." Gloss: As for: "A dislocation in a vertebra of his neck," he is speaking of a separation of one vertebra of his neck from another, the flesh which is over it being uninjured; as one says, "It is who," concerning things which had been joined together, when one has been severed from another.

Plato (428-348 BC)

First, then, the gods, imitating the spherical shape of the universe, enclosed the two divine courses in a spherical body, that, namely, which we now term the head, being the most divine part of us and the lord of all that is in us: to this the gods, when they put together the body, gave all the other members to be servants, considering that it partook of every sort of motion.

In order then that it might not tumble about among the high and deep places of the earth, but might be able to get over the one and out of the other, they provided the body to be its vehicle and means of locomotion; which consequently had length and was furnished with four limbs extended and flexible; these God contrived to be instrumnets of locomotion whith which it might take hold and find support, and so be able to pass through all places, carrying on high the dwelling place of the most sacred and divine part of us. Such was the origin of legs and hands, which for this reason were attached to every man.

Hippocrates (460-370 BC)

When, then, a dislocation has not been reduced, but has been misunderstood or neglected, the leg, in walking, is rolled about as is the case with oxen, and the weight of the body is mostly supported on the sound leg, and the limb at the flank, and the joint where the dislocation has occurred is necessarily hollow and bent, while on the sound side the buttock is necessarily rounded. For if one should walk with the foot of the sound leg turned outward, the weight of the body would be thrown upon the injured limb, but the injured limb could not carry it, for how could it? One, then, is forced in walking to turn the leg inward, and not outward, for thus the sound leg best supports its own half of the body, and also that of the injured side. But being hollow at the flank and the hip-joint, they appear small in stature, and are forced to rest on a staff at the side of the sound leg. For they require the support of a staff there, since the nates inclines to this side, and the weight of the body is carried to it. They are forced also to stoop, for they are obliged to rest the hand on the side of the thigh against the affected limb; for the limb which is injured cannot support the body in changing the legs, unless it be held when it is applied to the ground. They who have got an unreduced dislocation inward are forced to put themselves into these attitudes, and this from no premeditation on their part how they should assume the easiest position, but the impediment itself teaches them to choose that which is most conformable to their present circumstances. For persons who have a sore on the foot, or leg, and cannot rest upon the limb, all, even children, walk in this way; for they turn the injured limb outward in walking, and they derive two advantages there from, to supply two wants; the weight of the body is not equally thrown upon the limb turned outward, as upon the one turned inward, for neither is the weight in a line with it, but is much more thrown upon the one under the body; for the weight is in a straight line with it, both in walking and in the shifting of the legs. In this position one can most quickly turn the sound limb under the body, by walking with the unsound limb outward, and the sound inward. In the case we are now treating of, it is well that the body finds out the attitudes which are the easiest for itself. Those persons, then, who have not attained their growth at the time when they met with a dislocation which is not reduced, become maimed in the thigh, the leg, and the foot, for neither do the bones grow properly, but become shortened, and especially the bone of the thigh; and the whole limb is emaciated, loses its muscularity, and becomes enervated and thinner, both from the impediment at the joint, and because the patient cannot use the limb, as it does not lie in its natural position, for a certain amount of exercise will relieve excessive enervation, and it will remedy in so far the deficiency of growth in length. Those persons, then, are most maimed who have experienced the dislocation in utero, next those who have met with it in infancy, and least of all, those who are full grown. The mode of walking adopted by adults has been already described; but those who are children when this accident befalls them, generally lose the erect position of the body, and crawl about miserably on the sound leg, supporting themselves with the hand of the sound side resting on the ground. Some, also, who had attained manhood before they met with this accident, have also lost the faculty of walking erect. Those who were children when they met with the accident, and have been properly instructed, stand erect upon the sound leg, but carry about a staff, which they apply under the armpit of the sound side, and some use a staff in both arms; the unsound limb they bear up, and the smaller the unsound limb, the greater facility have they in walking, and their sound leg is no less strong than when both are sound. The fleshy parts of the limb are enervated in all such cases, but those who have dislocation inward are more subject to this loss of strength than, for the most part, those who have it outward.

When persons have attained their full growth before meeting with this dislocation, and when it has not been reduced, upon the subsidence of the pain, and when the bone of the joint has been accustomed to be rotated in the place where it is lodged, these persons can walk almost erect without a staff, and with the injured leg almost quite straight, as it does not admit of easy flexion at the groin and the ham; owing, then, to this want of flexion at the groin, they keep the limb more straight in walking than they do the sound one. And sometimes they drag the foot along the ground, as not being able to bend the upper part of the limb, and they walk with the whole foot on the ground; for in walking they rest no less on the heel than on the fore part of the foot; and if they could take great steps, they would rest entirely on the heel in walking; for persons whose limbs are sound, the greater the steps they take in walking, rest so much the more on the heel, while they are putting down the one foot and raising the opposite. In this form of dislocation, persons rest their weight more on the heel than on the anterior part of the foot, for the fore part of the foot cannot be bent forward equally well when the rest of the limb is extended as when it is in a state of flexion; neither, again, can the foot be arched to the same degree the limb is bent as when it is extended. The natural state of matters is such as has been now described; and in an unreduced dislocation, persons walk in the manner described, for the reasons which have been stated. The limb, moreover, is less fleshy than the other, at the nates, the calf of the leg, and the whole of its posterior part. When this dislocation occurs in infancy, and is not reduced, or when it is congenital, in these cases the bone of the thigh is more atrophied than those of the leg and foot; but the atrophy of the thigh-bone is least of all in this form of dislocation. The fleshy parts, however, are everywhere attenuated, more especially behind, as has been stated above. If properly trained, such persons, when they grow up, can use the limb, which is only a little shorter than the other, and yet they support themselves on a staff at the affected side. For, not being able to use properly the ball of the foot without the heel, nor to put it down as some can in the other varieties of dislocation (the cause of which has been just now stated), on this account they require a staff. But those who are neglected, and are not in the practice of putting their foot to the ground, but keep the limb up, have the bones more atrophied than those who use the limb; and, at the articulations, the limb is more maimed in the direct line than in the other forms of dislocation.

Aristotle (384-322 BC)

- what are the fewest points of motion necessary to animal progression
- why sanguineous animals have four points and not more, but bloodless animals more than four
- why some animals are footless, others bipeds, others quadrupeds, others polypods
- why all have an even number of feet
- why the points on which progression depends are even in number
- why are man and bird bipeds, but fish footless
- why do man and bird, though both bipeds, have an opposite curvature of the legs

Solutions

- the moving creature always changes its position by pressing against what lies below it (3)
- the beginning of movement is on the right: nature of the right is to initiate movement, that of the left to be moved
    - all men carry burdens on the left shoulder
    - hop easier on the left leg
    - all men lead off with the left
    - men guard themselves with their right
    - spiral-shaped Testaceans have their shells on the right, go forward in the direction opposite to the spire
    - all animals then start movement from the right

- the right is more dextrous than the left
- men and birds are biped because they have the superior part distinguished from the front (5)
- animals which have the superior and the front parts identically situated are four-footed, many-footed, or footless (6)
- the animal must act with opposite limbs, shifting the weight from the limbs that are being moved to those at rest (8)
- without flexion there could not be walking or swimming or flying (9)
- when then one leg is advanced it becomes the hypotenuse of a right-angled triangle (10)
    - its square then is equal to the square on the other side together with the square on the base
    - the one at rest must bend either at the knee
    - If a man were to walk parallel to a wall in sunshine, the line described (by the shadow of his head) would be not straight but zigzag, becoming lower as he bends, and higher when he stands and lifts himself up.
- birds are hunchbacked yet stand on two legs because their weight is set back (11)
    - their being bipeds and able to stand is above all due to their having the hip-bone shaped like a thigh
    - one in the leg before the knee-joint, the other joining his part to the fundament - not a thigh but a hip
- all creatures which naturally have the power of changing position by the use of limbs (12)
    - must have one leg stationary with the weight of the body on it
    - and when they move forward the leg which has the leading position must be unencumbered
    - and the progression continuing the weight must shift and be taken off on this leading leg
    - it is evidently necessary for the back leg from being bent to become straight again
    - while the point of movement of the leg thrust forward and its lower part remain still
- bird though a biped is not erect, and has the forward parts of the body lighter than the hind (15)

Archimedes (287-212 BC)

Another Greek, determined hydrostatic principles governing floating bodies that are still accepted as swimming. In addition, Heath (1972) suggests that his inquiries included the laws of leverage and determining the center of gravity and the foundation of the oretical mechanics.

Galen (131-201 AD)

Roman citizen who tended the Pergamum's gladiators in Asia Minor and is considered to have been the first team physician in history.

He used number to describe muscles. His essay De Motu Musculorum (On the Movements of Muscles) distinguished between motor and sensory nerves, agonist and antagonist muscles, described tonus, and introduced terms such as diarthrosis and synarthrosis.

He taught that muscular contraction resulted from the passage of "animal spirits" from the brain through the nerves to the muscles. Snook (1978) suggested that some writers consider his treatise the first textbook on kinesiology, and he has been termed "the father of sports medicine." Due to his era's discouragement of human dissection, the majority of Galen's work was based on the dissections of dogs, pigs, and apes.

The Renaissance

Leonardo da Vinci (1452-1519)

This artist, engineer, and scientist, da Vinci was particularly interested in the structure of the human body as it relates to performance, center of gravity and the balance and center of resistance.

He used letter to identify muscles and nerves in the human body that he retrived from grave yards in the middle ofthe night. ( ) He described the mechanics of the body during standing, walking up and downhill, rising from a sitting position, jumping, and human gait.

To demonstrate the progressive action and interaction ofvarious muscles during movement, he suggested that cords be attached to a skeleton at the points oforigin and insertion of the muscles.

Galileo Galilei (1564-1642)

Galileo Galilei was a student of medicine before he became famous as a physicist. He discovered the constancy of the pediod of a pendulum, and used the pendulum to measure the pulse rate of people, expressing the results quantitatively in terms of the lenght of a pendulum syncronous to the heart.

Galielo's fame was so grea and his lectures in Padua so popular that his influence on biomechanics went far beyond his personal contribtions. According to Singer (History, p. 237), William Harvey should be regarded a disciple of Galileo. Harvey studied in Padua (1598-1601) while Galileo was active there. By 1615 Harvey had formed the concept of circulation of blood. He published his demonstration in 1628. The essential part of his demonstration is the result not of mere observation but of the application of Galieleo's principle of measurement. He showed first thatthe blood can only leave the ventricle of the heart in one direction. Then he measured the capacity of the heart, and found it to be about two ounces. The heart beats 72 times a minute, so that in one hour it throws into the system 2x72x60 ounces =8640 ounces = 234 kg! Where can all this blood come from? Where can it all go? He concludes that the existence of circuation is a necessary condition for the function of the heart.

Giovani Alfonso Borelli (1608-1679)

Eminent Italian mathematician and astronomer, and a friend of Galieleo. His On the Motion of Animals (De Motu Animalum) 1680 is a classic. He was succesful in clarifying muscular movement and body dynamics. He treated the flight of birds and the swimming of fish, as well as the movement of the heart and the intestines.

Borelli estimated the center of mass of nude men by having them stretch out on a rigid platform supported on a knife edge. The platform was then repositioned until is balanced, thereby indicating a location corresponding to the center of mass for the entire body.

William Croone (1633-1684)

Studied the process by which signals from the brain cause a muscle contraction.

Luigi Galvani (1737-1798)

During the summer of 1786 studied the effects of atmospheric electricity on dissected frog muscles. He observed that the muscles of a frog sometimes contracted when touched by a scalpel, which led him to the conclusion that there was "in dwelling electricity which proceeded along the nerve." His Commentary on thr Effects of Electricity on Muscular Motion (1791) is probably the earliest explicit statement of the presence of electrical potentials in nerve and muscle. Galvani is considered the father of experimental neurology.

Basic Biomechanical Terms

The Description of Motion

1.1 Mass

The quantity of matter in an object. Mass can be thought of conceptually as the number of atoms in the object that would, of course, remain constant regardless of location or gravitational conditions (e.g., earth or moon gravity). Weight, however, would vary under these two conditions. The importance of mass in mechanics is that it represents, in linear terms, the resistance to a change of state (a speeding up or slowing down).

Note:	See discussion of confusion between the pound as a unit of both force and mass in 9.3.
Units:	SI—kilogram (kg)
	US Customary—pound mass (lbm)
Symbol:	m (or spell out with first use to avoid confusion with abbreviation for meter if context is not clear)

1.2 Rigid Body

A collection of particles occupying fixed locations with respect to each other. The assumption is that a rigid body will not deform under the action of an applied force however large the force may be. Obviously, this is an approximation in every case because all known materials deform by some amount under the action of a force (See 6.6). Nevertheless, the assumption that segments of the human body are rigid is used in almost every whole body biomechanical analysis that has been published to date (See Section 8).

1.3 Center of Mass

The point on a body that moves in the same way that a particle subject to the same external forces would move. Examples of the location of the center of mass of the human body in two different positions are shown in Figure 1.

Note: The center of mass is not necessarily located in the body as Figure 1 shows.

Synonym: first moment of mass, center of gravity (See 1.4)

Symbol: C of M, COM

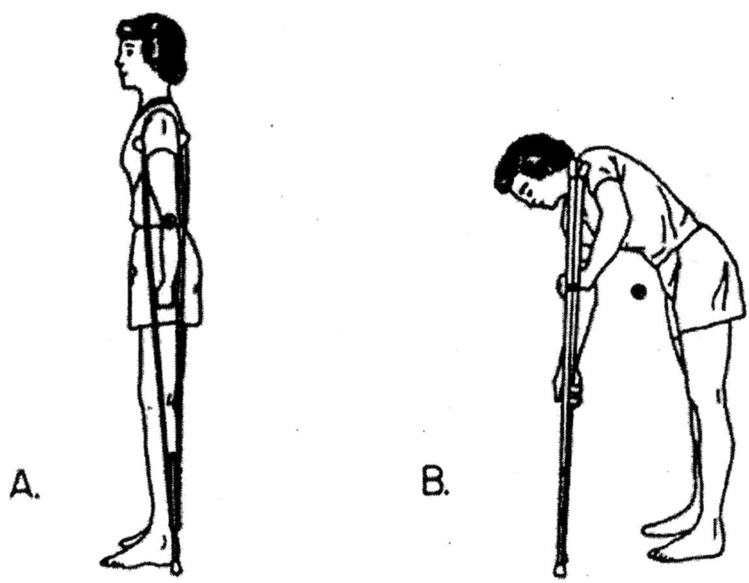

Figure 1. The location of the whole body center of mass (indicated by the circled cross) in two different postures A. center of mass is inside the body and B. center of mass is outside the body.

1.4 Center of Gravity

The point at which a single force of magnitude mg—mass times gravity—(the weight of the body or system) should be applied to a rigid body or system to balance exactly the translational and rotational effects of gravitational forces acting on the components of the body or system. In other words, the point at which the weight of the body or system can be considered to act.

Note: i. For all practical purposes, the center of gravity and the center of mass are coincident, although in strict physical terms, there is an infinitesimal difference between the two.

ii. The center of gravity of the human body is not fixed at an anatomical location. Its location varies according to the position of the body segments.

Synonym: center of mass (not necessarily located in the body as Figure 1 shows) but not center of pressure (See 2.17).

Symbol: C of G, COG

1.5 Moment of Inertia

The rotational equivalent of mass in its mechanical effect, that is, the resistance to a change of state (a speeding up or slowing down) during rotation. Intuitively, this would appear to be dependent on the mass of the object and the way the mass is distributed. In fact, the effect of distribution of mass is dominant as the following formula indicates:

$$I = m \cdot r^2 \qquad (1)$$

where m = mass and r = distance from axis of rotation.

Note: Unlike mass, for which there is only one value, a new value exists for moment of inertia for each new axis that is chosen.

Units: SI—kilogram meter squared ($kg \cdot m^2$)

US Customary—slug inch squared ($sl \cdot in^2$)

Synonym: second moment of mass

Symbol: I_{kk} where kk represents the axis about which the moment of inertia is calculated

1.6 Radius of Gyration

An abstract concept sometimes used for the estimation of moment of inertia of body segments. If all the mass in a rigid body were assumed to be concentrated at one point located a distance k from the axis of rotation kk such that $m \cdot k^2$ equals I_{kk}, then the distance k is said to equal the radius of gyration.

Because

$$m \cdot k^2 = I_{kk} \quad (2)$$

$$k = SQRT(I_{kk}/m) \quad (3)$$

Symbol – k

Units – same as units of displacement

1.7 Linear Motion

Motion in which all parts of the body travel along parallel paths.

Note: This does not imply motion in a straight line that is known as rectilinear translation. Linear motion along a curved path (curvilinear translation) is possible as long as the body does not rotate.

Synonym: translation

1.8 Angular Motion

Motion that is not linear. If the axis of rotation is fixed, all particles in the body travel in a circular manner. If the axis of rotation is not fixed the motion is actually a combination of translation and rotation.

Note: The motion of many limb segments is assumed to occur about fixed axes, although the joint centers do in fact migrate.

Units: SI—radians (rad, do not abbreviate if context is not clear)

US Customary—degrees (°) (deg), revolution (rev)

1.9 Scalar

A quantity that only has magnitude. For example, mass, length, or kinetic energy are scalar quantities and can be manipulated with conventional arithmetic.

1.10 Vector

A quantity that has both direction and magnitude. A force, for example, is always described by how big it is and by the direction in which it is acting. Velocity is also a vector quantity because it expresses the rate of change of position in a given direction.

Note: When performing calculations with vectors, ordinary arithmetic will give the wrong answers; therefore, vector addition and other types of vector algebra must be used. For example, the net effect of forces of 50 and 100 N acting at 90 degrees to each other is actually 111.8 N acting at 63 degrees to the 50 N vector (Fig . 2). In equations of motion, a vector quantity will always contribute two unknowns—one for magnitude and one for direction.

Symbol: a, ā, a, (length and direction depend on the given vector)

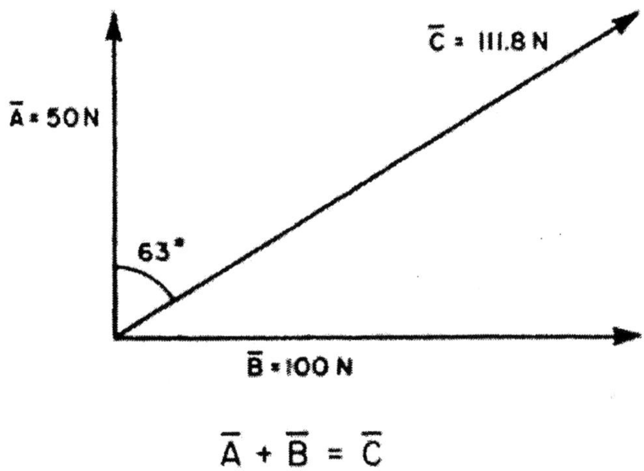

Figure 2. Vector addition. The sum of vector quantities A and B is vector C. Use either mathematics or geometry (the parallelogram rule) to find the sum.

1.11 Displacement

The change in the position of a body. This change may be translational, whereby every point of the body is displaced along parallel lines; it may be rotational, with the points of the body describing concentric circles around an axis; or it may be a combination of the two. For example, although the general movement of the human body during locomotion is translational, the limbs act with rotatory motion around many joints to obtain this end result.

Units: SI—linear: meters (m); rotational: radians

US Customary—linear: feet (ft); rotational: degrees (°) (deg) or revolutions (rev).

Symbol: x or s

1.12 Velocity

A measure of a body's motion in a given direction. Because velocity has both magnitude and direction, it is a vector quantity that can be positive, negative, or zero. Linear velocity is the rate at which a body moves in a straight line. Mathematically, velocity is the first derivative with respect to time of displacement (See 4.4) and the first integral with respect to time of acceleration (See 4.6).

Note: i. The velocity is dependent on which reference frame is used in the computation (See 4.8). For example, the calculation of relative velocity of one body with respect to another uses reference frames that move with both bodies.

ii. Because velocity is a vector quantity, it can be expressed as components in any direction, such as horizontally and vertically.

Units: SI—meters/second (m/s)

US Customary—feet/second (ft/sec or ft/s), miles per hour (mph)

Synonym: Speed and velocity are not synonyms. Speed is a scalar quantity that designates rate and not direction.

Symbol: v,υ

1.13 Angular Velocity

The rate of movement in rotation calculated as the first time derivative of angular displacement.

Note: Like linear velocity, angular velocity can be expressed in terms of components along the axes of a coordinate system.

Units: SI—radians/sec (rad/s)

US Customary—revolutions/min (rpm), degrees/sec (° /sec) (° /s) (deg/sec)

Note on units: Sometimes the units of angular velocity are given units: as sec^{-1} because all the measures of angle are dimensionless (See 9.4).

Symbol: ω (omega)

1.14 Acceleration

The rate of change of velocity with respect to time, mathematically the second time derivative of displacement and the first time derivative of velocity (See 4.4). Acceleration is also a vector quantity that may take positive, negative, or zero values.

Note: The term "deceleration" is redundant because it is simply negative acceleration. Note that it is entirely possible to have positive velocity and negative acceleration and the reverse.

Units: SI—meters per second per second (m/s^2)

US Customary—feet per second per second or inches per second per second (ft/sec^2 or in/sec^2) (ft/s^2 or in/s^2)

Symbol: a

1.15 Angular Acceleration

Angular acceleration refers to the rate at which the angular velocity of a body changes with respect to time. In algebraic form, average angular acceleration is equal to the final angular velocity minus the initial angular velocity divided by the time taken.

Units: SI—radians per second per second (radian/s^2)

US Customary—revolutions per second per second (rev/sec^2) (rev/s^2) or degrees per second per second (° /sec^2 or deg/sec^2 or ° /s^2)

Symbols: α

SECTION 2 FORCES

2.1 Force

A vector quantity that describes the action of one body on another. The action may be direct, such as the foot pressing on the floor, or it may be indirect, such as the gravitational attraction between the body and the earth. Force can never be measured directly. It is always estimated, for example, by measuring the deflection of a spring under the action of a force.

Units: SI—newton (N)

US Customary—pound force (lbf)

Symbol: F

2.2 Resultant Force

At any one time, many forces may be acting on a body. The resultant force is the result obtained when all the forces acting are added vectorially (See 4.7) and expressed as a single force.

Units: SI—newton (N)

US Customary—pound force (lbf)

Synonym: net force

Symbol: F_r

2.3 Equilibrium

That condition when the resultant force and moment acting on a body are zero.

Note: This does not imply that the body is at rest or that there are no forces acting on the body.

2.4 Moment Arm

The perpendicular distance from the point of application of a force to the axis of rotation.

Synonym: lever arm

2.5 Moment

The turning effect produced by a force. Calculated as the product of the force and the perpendicular distance between the point of application of the force and the axis of rotation. In vector terms, the calculation is the vector (cross) product of force and distance.

Units: SI—newton meters (N · m)

US Customary—pound force feet (lbf · ft)

Note: These units have the same dimensions as those for work, and the context should be used to distinguish between the two quantities.

Synonym: torque (but some controversy exists on this point)

Symbol: M

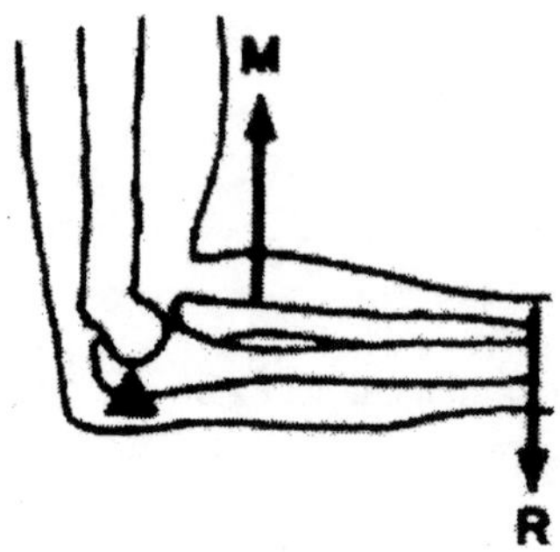

Third Class Level

Figure 3. Examples of the three classes of levers (adapted from LeVeau[1]). The fulcrum is indicated by the solid triangle. M represents muscle force, and R represents resisting force.

2.8 Mechanical Advantage

The mechanical advantage of a lever system is the ratio of the effort-force lever arm to the resisting-force lever arm. A ratio of 1 indicates no change in mechanical advantage, less than 1 a decrease, and greater than 1 an increase in mechanical advantage. A first-class lever can therefore have any value for mechanical advantage, a second class lever always has a value greater than 1, and a third-class lever always has a value less than 1.

Symbol: MA

2.9 Weight

The force that results from the action of a gravitational field on a mass. Weight can be thought of as the force an object exerts on a stationary supporting surface placed perpendicular to a gravitational field (and by Newton's third law as the force the surface exerts on the object).

Note: When we "weigh" ourselves, we are determining weight not mass, but as long as the gravitational field is the same (the acceleration resulting from gravity does not change), mass can be estimated from weight using Newton's second law.

Units: SI—newton (N)

US Customary—pound force (lbf)

Synonym: none (especially not mass) but weight is equal to the ground reaction force when the object is at rest on a horizontal surface

Symbol: W (or spell out to avoid confusion with abbreviation for work or watt if context is not clear)

2.10 Friction

The tangential force acting between two bodies in contact that opposes motion or impending motion. If the two bodies are at rest, then the frictional forces are called static friction. If there is relative motion between the two bodies, then the forces acting between the surfaces are called kinetic friction. Two types of friction exist: dry fiction, also called coulomb friction, and fluid friction. Most biomechanical analyses involve dry friction. The maximum force of static friction between any pair of dry unlubricated surfaces follows two laws: 1) it is independent of the contact area, and 2) it is proportional to the normal force. The normal force is exerted by either body on the other, perpendicular to their mutual interface. The ratio of the magnitude of static friction to the magnitude of the normal force is called the coefficient of static friction and shows the following relationship: $f = \mu_s N$, where f = friction, μ_s = coefficient of static friction, and N (in this case) = magnitude of the normal force.

Units: SI—newton (N)

US Customary—pound force (lbf)

Symbol: f for the frictional force and μ_s for the coefficient of friction.

2.11 Joint Forces

The forces that exist between the articular surfaces of the joint. Joint forces are the result of muscle forces, gravity, and inertial forces (usually, muscle forces are responsible for the largest part).[2]

Units: SI—newton (N)

US Customary—pound force (lbf)

Synonym: bone on bone forces but not joint reaction forces

2.12 Joint Reaction Forces

The equal and opposite forces that exist between adjacent bones at a joint caused by the weight and inertial forces of the two segments. Joint reaction force is a fairly abstract concept useful in mathematical analysis but not much use in practice. This quantity must not be confused with joint forces that include the effects of muscle action.[2]

Units: SI—newton (N)

US Customary—pound force (lbf)

Synonym: none but not joint forces or bone on bone forces

2.13 Ground Reaction Forces

The forces that act on the body as a result of interaction with the ground.[3] Newton's third law implies that ground reaction forces are equal and opposite to those that the body is applying to the ground. Ground reaction forces can be measured with a force platform.

Notes: i. The conventions usually adopted are those shown in Figure 4, where positive forces act in the following manner:

F_x Horizontally tending to push the foot laterally.

F_y Horizontally tending to push the foot backwards.

F_z Vertically upwards.

ii. The above three directions do not constitute a right-handed Cartesian system (See 4.14). This is because the forces were originally defined not as ground reaction forces but as forces applied to the platform that are, by Newton's third law,' equal and opposite to the ground reaction forces. This system is also shown in Figure 4.

The choice to use either ground reaction forces or forces applied to the platform is a fundamental one that must be made depending on the particular study.

Units: SI—newton (N)

US Customary—pound force (lbf)

2.14 Inertial Forces

The product of the mass of a body and its acceleration or the moment of inertia and the angular acceleration.

Note: A system of drawing free body diagrams referred to as D'Alembert's theorem involves adding inertial forces to the free body diagram. This method is not recommended.

Synonym: inertia forces

2.15 Gravitational Force

The force exerted on an object as a result of gravitational pull. This force may be considered as a single force representing the sum of all the individual weights within the object.

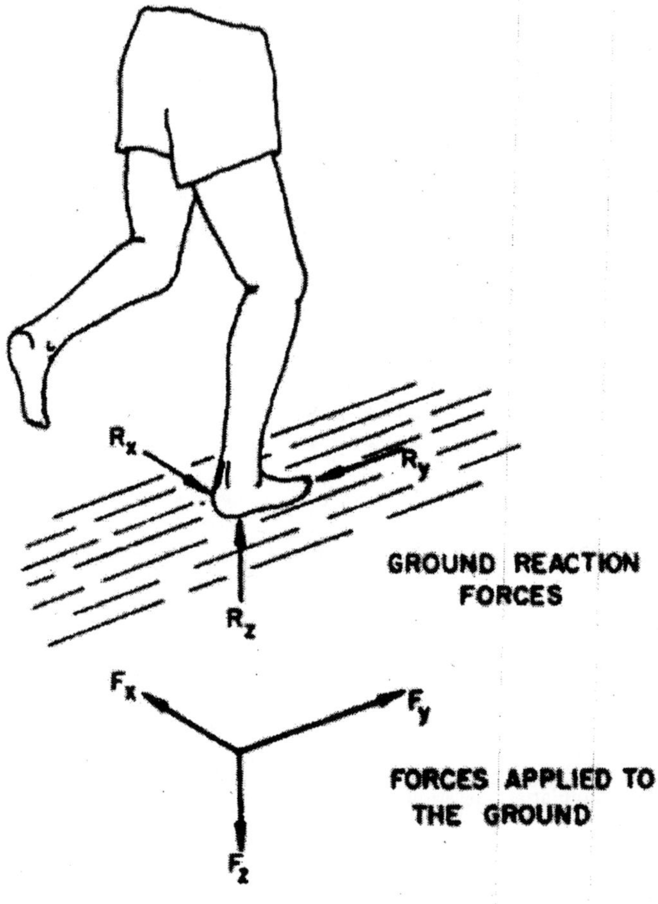

Figure 4. Usual conventions for the effect of ground reaction forces on the body: positive Fx—lateral (to both feet), positive Fy—backwards, positive Fz—upward.

2.16 g

The symbol used to represent the acceleration because of gravity on earth. Although this quantity actually varies according to location and altitude, the usual value used is 9.81 m/sec^2 (or 32.2 ft/sec^2), which is the value measure in Paris, France.

Note:	The symbol is sometimes used incorrectly as a synonym for acceleration.
Units:	SI—meters per second squared (m/s^2)
	US Customary—feet per second squared (ft/sec^2) (ft/s^2)
Synonym:	not G (which stands for the Universal Constant of Gravitation)
Symbol:	g

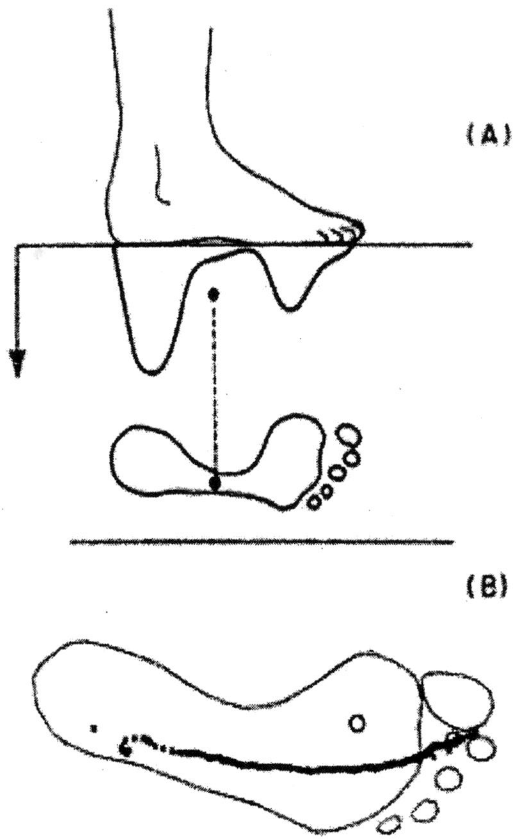

2.17 Center of Pressure

A quantity available from a force platform describing the centroid of the pressure distribution (Fig. 5).[3] It can be thought of as (and is sometimes called) the point of application of the force, but this is a somewhat misleading definition unless the force is truly applied at a point (e.g., by the tip of a walking cane). In the more general case, the force is applied over a diffuse area (e.g., the plantar aspect of the foot).

Units: SI—meters (m) (or relative units—e.g., % of foot length from heel origin)

US Customary—feet (ft)

Synonym: point of force application, force line origin

Symbols: The x, y coordinates are sometimes referred to as CPX, CPY in the ground reaction force reference frame shown in Figure 4.

Figure 5. The meaning of center of pressure (C of P). A theoretical distribution of pressure during standing (A). When pressure exists under both the heel and ball of the foot, the C of P will be in the midfoot region, which in itself is not bearing much pressure. During walking, the C of P can be plotted as it moves under the foot (B).

2.18 Force Line

A line representing the resultant ground reaction force vector drawn starting at the center of pressure and with magnitude and direction determined by the measured components of the ground reaction force vector. This presentation has become more relevant recently because hardware devices are available to combine force platform and video outputs to display the force line immediately after a patient has been examined.

Note: See 2.17, limitations on the meaning of the center of pressure, which is where the force line originates.

Units: If the video display has both sagittal and frontal views the force line presentation contains five distinct pieces of information and, therefore, the units need a scale for each that should appear on the display.

CPX—center of pressure X coordinate—meters

(or % shoe or foot length)

CPY—center of pressure Y coordinate—meters

(or % shoe or foot length)

F_z—vertical component of GRF—N (newtons)

F_y—anteroposterior component of GRF—N

(newtons)

F_x—mediolateral component of GRF—N (newtons)

A sagittal view will contain only F_y, F_z, and CPY.

KINETICS— the Study of the Forces that Cause Motion

3.1 Newton's Laws

Three laws that form the basis of conventional or Newtonian Mechanics. The laws can be remembered by the acronym IN-MO-RE: 1) first law of INertia, 2) second law of MOmentum, and 3) third law of REaction.

Newton's first law states that a body will maintain a state of rest or uniform motion unless acted on by a net force.

Newton's second law states that the change in momentum of the body under the action of a resultant force will be proportional to the product of the magnitude of the force and the time for which it acts (i.e., the impulse). The second law also states that the change in momentum will be in the direction of the resultant force.

Newton's third law states that action and reaction are equal and opposite. Although the first and third laws are somewhat intuitive, the second law provides a means for 1) the formulation of equations of motion (See 4.11), 2) the definition of units of force (See Section 9, and Section 3) the formulation of the impulse momentum relationship (See 3.5). The second law is frequently stated as, "Force equals mass times acceleration" ($F = m \cdot a$). This is derived from the formal statement of the law using the following symbols:

v_1 = initial velocity (before force starts to act)

v_2 = final velocity (after force has acted)

m = mass of object

F = magnitude of a constant force

t = time for which force acts

a = average acceleration

$$\text{Change in momentum} = mv_2 - mv_1 \quad (4)$$

$$\text{impulse} = \text{force x time} = F \cdot t \quad (5)$$

therefore,

$$F \cdot t = mv_2 - mv_1 \quad (6)$$

then,

$$F = m(v_2 - v_1)/t \quad (7)$$

but,

$$(v_2 - v_1)/t = \text{acceleration.} \quad (8)$$

Therefore,

$$F = m \cdot a \quad (9)$$

Thus, the second law can be restated as, "The force acting on a body is equal to the mass of the body multiplied by its acceleration." The definition of units of force follows directly from this statement of the law (See Section 9).

3.2 Impulse

The effect of a force acting over a period of time. Impulse is determined mathematically by the integral of the force-time curve, more simply thought of as the area under the force-time curve. Newton's second law allows us to quantify the effect of a force on the velocity of an object if we know the impulse by the impulse-momentum relationship.

Units: SI—newton seconds that reduce to kg · m/s (N · s)

US Customary—pound force seconds (lbf · s) (lbf · sec)

3.3 Linear Momentum

The product of the mass of an object and its linear velocity.

Note: The units are the same as those for impulse as is necessary for the impulse-momentum relationship to be dimensionally homogeneous (See 9.4).

Units: SI—kilogram meters per sec (kg · m/s)

US Customary—foot pounds per sec (lb · ft/sec) (lb ft/s)

3.4 Angular Momentum

The rotational equivalent of linear momentum that can be thought of as describing the "amount of motion" that the body possesses during rotation. Computationally, it is the product of the moment of inertia and the angular velocity (angular momentum = I_{kk})

Note: Because angular momentum is a vector quantity, it can be resolved into components. It is possible to have angular momentum about one axis and none about another. Angular momentum can, however, be transferred from one axis to another.

Units: SI—kilogram meters squared per sec ($kg \cdot m^2/s$)

US Customary—pound feet squared per sec ($lb \cdot ft^2/sec$) ($lb \cdot ft^2/s$)

Symbol: H (or spell out to avoid confusion with abbreviation for henry if context is not clear)

3.5 Impulse-Momentum Relationship

The change in momentum experienced by a body under the action of a force is equal to the impulse of the resultant force. This follows directly from the definition of Newton's second law.

3.6 Work

Work is done when a force moves an object through a distance. Whenever a constant force exists and motion takes place in a straight line, then work equals the magnitude of the force (F) times the distance (d) through which the object moves: $W = F \cdot d$. If the force is not constant, work equals the integral of force with respect to distance:

$$W = \int F\,dx \qquad (1)$$

Notes:

i. According to this definition, no mechanical work is done during isometric action of a muscle. An ongoing debate about the implications of this exists because any muscle action clearly involves the expenditure of metabolic energy.

ii. The definition of work is independent of time.

Thus, the same amount of work is done in raising a 20 kg weight overhead slowly or quickly. The power in these situations is not, however, the same (See 3.7).

Unit: SI—joule (J)

US Customary—foot pound (ft · lbf)

Symbol: W (which is also the abbreviation for the SI unit of power—the watt, and for weight)

3.7 Power

The rate of doing work- Power is equal to the work done divided by the time during which the work is being done: P = W/t. More strictly, this definition is "average power" because it is possible to calculate the "instantaneous power" by taking the derivative of work as a function of time: P = dW/dt.

Unit: SI—watt (W)

US Customary—horsepower (hp) or foot pound per second (ft.· lb/sec)

Synonym: Work rate (but this is colloquial and should not be used)

Symbol: P

3.8 Energy

The capacity for doing work. In any system, this capacity cannot be destroyed, but energy can be transformed from one form to another (this is a statement of the Principle of Conservation of Energy). In biomechanics, the forms of energy that are most frequently encountered are kinetic energy, potential energy, strain energy, and heat energy.

Note: The units of work and energy are the same

because of the relationship of these two quantities through the work-energy principle (See 3.11).

Units: SI—joule (J)

US Customary—foot pound (ft · lb)

Symbol: E

Synonym: Although work and energy are closely related, they should not be used synonymously. The context should be used to determine the correct usage.

3.9 Kinetic Energy

That component of the mechanical energy of a body resulting from its motion. Two forms of kinetic energy are identified.

Kinetic energy of translation = ½ $m \cdot v^2$ (11)

Kinetic energy of rotation = ½ $I_{kk} \cdot \omega^2$ (12)

Units: SI—joule (J)

US Customary—foot pound (ft · lb)

Symbol: T, however, KE is more commonly used TKE is used for translational kinetic energy RKE is used for rotational kinetic energy

3.10 Potential Energy

That component of the mechanical energy of a body resulting from its position.

$$\text{Potential Energy} = m \cdot g \cdot h \qquad (13)$$

where m is mass, g is acceleration resulting from gravity, and h is distance above datum (see note below).

Units: SI—joule (J)

US Customary—foot pound (ft · lb)

Note: Potential energy is always calculated according to an arbitrary reference point or datum and can therefore assume any value depending on the choice of the datum. This is not as impractical as it seems because it is frequently the change in potential energy that is important and this is independent of the choice of a datum.

Symbol: V, however, PE is more commonly used (V is also used as an abbreviation for volt)

3.11 Work-Energy Principle

The work done on a body is equal to the change of kinetic energy of the body. A more comprehensive statement is that the work done on the body is equal to the change in the energy level of the body.

Note: If the change in E_{tot} is positive, then work has been done on the body—positive work. If the change in E_{tot} is negative, then the body has done work on some other body—negative work.

3.12 Energy Level

The total mechanical energy of a body or system. This total represents the sum of the translational and rotational kinetic energy and the potential energy.

$$\text{Energy level} = KET + KER + PE \qquad (14)$$

$$E_{tot} = (\frac{1}{2} m \cdot v^2) + (\frac{1}{2} I_{kk} \cdot \omega^2) + (m \cdot g \cdot h) \qquad (15)$$

Note — Some published work has attempted to equate the changes in energy levels of all segments of the body with the expenditure of metabolic energy. Although these quantities are dimensionally homogeneous (See 9.4), a number of biological reasons exist why this relationship is inexact (See 5.10).

Units: SI—joule (J)

US Customary—foot pound (ft · lb)

Synonym: total mechanical energy

Symbol: E_{tot}

SECTION 4 COMPUTATIONAL METHODS

4.1 Composition of Vectors

The use of vector algebra to combine vectors that act in the same plane (coplanar) and that have the same point of application (concurrent). The use of vector algebra to combine vectors in this way is called composition of vectors. An example of this is shown in Figure 2.

Synonym: vector addition

4.2 Resolution of Vectors

The reverse process from vector composition. One approach to writing equations of motion involves the derivation of both horizontal and vertical equations. Because vectors will not, in general, act in either of these directions, one vector is resolved (Figure 6) using vector algebra into two components that are in the required directions.

Synonym: taking components

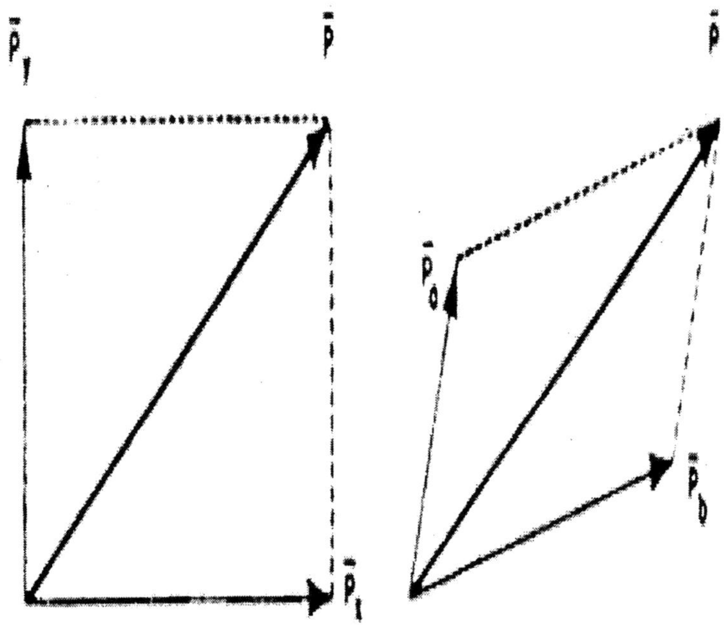

Figure 6. Resolution of vectors using a parallelogram method. The vector P can be resolved into two or more components in any chosen directions, such as Py and Px or Pa and Pd.

4.3 Differentiation

A technique of calculus for finding the rate of change of a quantity. This can result in a single value (for the instantaneous rate of change) or a new curve derived from the rate of change at each point. Graphically, the process can be thought of as determining the instantaneous gradient of a curve (the change in the y-direction divided by the change in the x-direction), assuming conventional Cartesian axes and coordinates (See 4.14). Differentiation can be performed graphically (by drawing tangents to the curve), numerically (by calculating the difference between two adjacent y values divided by the difference between the x values of the same points), or analytically (according to a set of rules for functions such as $y = ax^2 + bx + c$).

Note: i. The quantities do not necessarily vary with time, but they can be functions of any variable (e.g., distance).

ii. Differentiation of an unsmoothed signal (e.g., the output of an electrogoniometer) can produce almost meaningless data because the process is biased in favor of high frequency components that are often present as "noise" in the data (See 4.12). Similar comments apply to differentiation of numerical data collected from film analysis using a digitizer. Therefore, some form of filtering (See 4.13) almost always precedes differentiation.

Symbol: d(a)/db, where a is being differentiated with respect to b. Note that a and b would be on the x- and y-axes of a conventional plot.

4.4 Derivatives

Quantities obtained by the process of differentiating a given curve or function. The most commonly used derivatives are of displacement (x) where first derivatives dx/dt = velocity, second derivative d^2x/dt^2 = acceleration, and third derivative d^3x/dt^3 = jerk.

Note: Acceleration is obtained from jerk, velocity from acceleration, and displacement from velocity by the reverse process (integration).

4.5 Integration

A technique of calculus for determining the area enclosed between a curve and the x-axis. This can result in either a single value or a new curve derived from the varying function. Integration can be performed either graphically, mathematically, or numerically, and it is the inverse process of differentiation.

Notes: i. Unlike differentiation, integration tends to be a

smoothing process and, therefore, the curve obtained from integration is smoother than the one from which it was derived.

ii. Limits of integration establish where on the x-axis of the curve, the integration is to be started and terminated.

iii. Initial conditions are needed to evaluate completely an integral (called a definite integral). Typically, if a body was at rest before a force began to act, the initial condition would be v = 0 at t = 0.

Symbol: $_{LL}\int^{UL}$a db, where a is on the y-axis of a conventional plot, b is on the x-axis of a conventional plot, LL is the lower limit of b at which integration is to be started, and UL is the upper limit of b at which integration is to be ended.

4.6 Integrals

Quantities obtained by the process of integration. In biomechanics some of the most commonly used integrals are velocity = integral of acceleration with respect to time, displacement = integral of velocity with respect to time, and work = integral of power with respect to time.

4.7 Vector Algebra

A set of definitions, rules, and operations used for computational purposes in the manipulation of vector quantities. The two most well-known operations are

vector (or cross) product = A x B = AB cos(θ) (16)

scalar (or dot) product = A · B = |A| |B| sin(θ) (17)

where A and B are vectors and θ is the angle between them. The symbol | | means the magnitude (size) of the enclosed quantity regardless of sign. The multiplication of A and B in the vector product involves a multiplication of all the components of the two vectors using matrix algebra. The multiplication of the magnitudes of A and B in the scalar product is conventional multiplication of two numbers. The physical result of the vector product is a third vector mutually perpendicular to A and B (Fig. 7) and the result of a scalar product is a scalar that represents the size of the projection of vector A and vector B (Fig. 8). Resolution and composition of vectors are further examples of vector algebra.

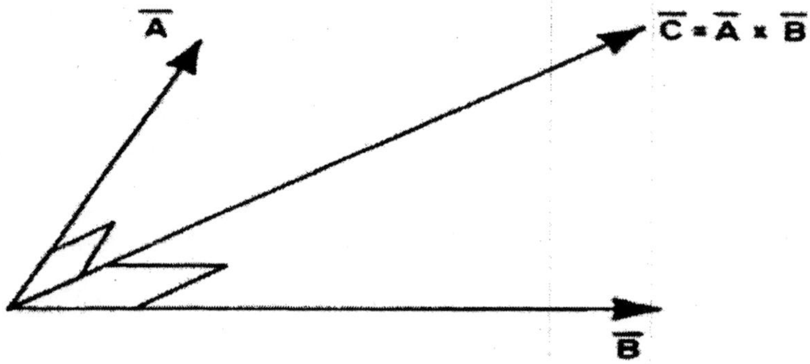

Figure 7. The vector product of vectors A and B is a vector that is perpendicular to both and is physically represented here as vector C

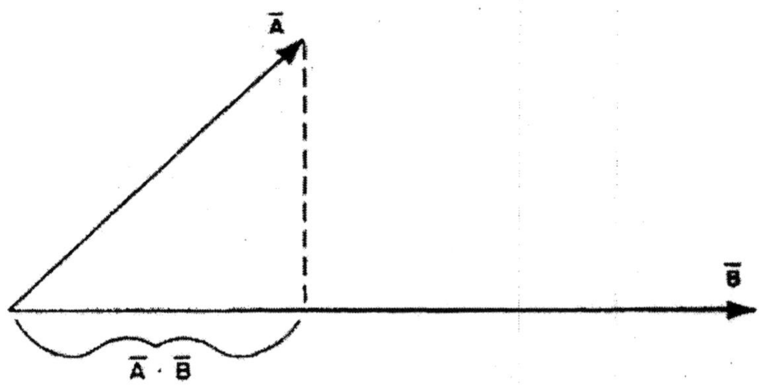

Figure. 8. The vector C, the result of the scalar product A · B, represents the projection of vector A on vector B.

4.8 Reference Frame

An origin and a set of coordinate axes that serve as the basis for the calculation of displacement and its derivatives. Many types of reference frames are frequently used.

a. Inertial reference frames: Reference frames that are fixed relative to the space in which objects are moving. Inertial reference frames are, in general, reference frames fixed in the earth. The term "fixed reference frames" is sometimes used as a synonym, but this is incorrect because all reference frames are fixed to some point even if the point happens to be moving.

b. Moving reference frames: Reference frames that are "body fixed' and move with the body being studied. The use of moving reference frames allows the spatial relationships between two objects to be expressed using matrix algebra but also introduces other complications (See 4.14).

Symbols: oXY in two dimensions where o is the origin and X and Y are the rectangular coordinate axes

oXYZ in three dimensions where Z is the third axis

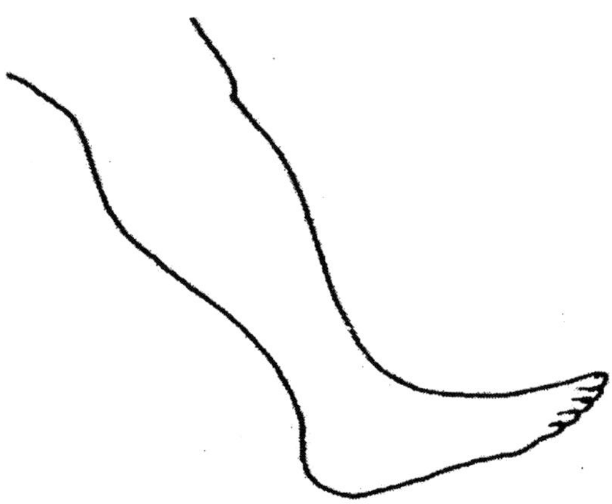

Figure 9. Space diagram of a lower leg during the swing phase of gait.

4.9 Space Diagrams

A representation of an object in the environment in which it is to be studied. This diagram should include other bodies and surfaces that the object contacts. An example is shown in Figure 9.

4.10 Free Body Diagram

A diagram in which all the forces and torques acting on a body are identified. This includes forces like gravity, frictional forces, and reaction forces caused by contact with other objects. The name originates from the fact that the body is "freed" from its external contacts that are replaced by reaction forces. The drawing of a free body diagram is an essential first step to the solution of problems in statics and dynamics. A free body diagram for the same situation demonstrated in the space diagram of Figure 9 is shown in Figure 10.

Symbol: FBD

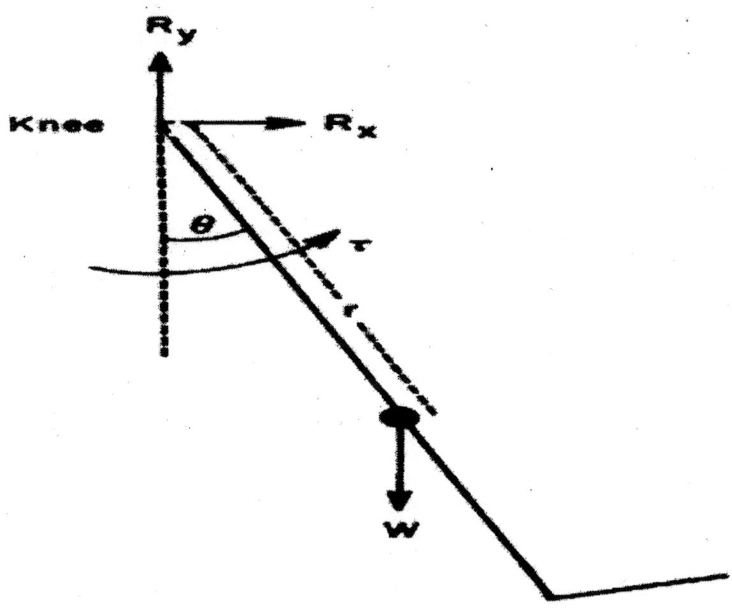

Figure 10. Free body diagram of the lower leg in the swing phase of gait. Rx and Ry = joint reaction forces: W = segment weight; θ = segment angle; T (tau) = joint moment; r = distance to segment C of G.

4.11 Equations of Motion

Equations obtained by using Newton's second law to equate, in the linear case, the resultant force acting on a body with the product of the linear accelerations and the mass. In the angular case, the relationship is between the net moment acting on a body and the product of moment of inertia and angular acceleration. The equations are usually written following the drawing of a free body diagram in which all the forces and moments acting on the body are identified. The equations of motion for the free body diagram given in Figure 10 are shown in Figure 11.

Vertical

$$R_y - W = \frac{W}{g}\ddot{y}$$

Horizontal

$$R_x = \frac{W}{g}\ddot{x}$$

Rotational

$$\tau - R_x r \cos\theta - R_y r \sin\theta - I_{CG}\ddot{\theta} = 0$$

Figure 11. Equations of motion for the free body diagram shown in Figure 10. Where x and y = components of acceleration in x and y directions; I_{cg} = moment of inertia of segment about C of G; θ = angular acceleration; Rx and Ry = joint reaction forces; W = segment weight; θ = segment angle; T (tau) = joint moment; r = distance to segment C of G.

4.12 Noise

Error present in data collected that is unrelated to the process being studied. Some noise is almost always present in data collected in biomechanics and most other fields.

Some typical examples are noise caused by human error in digitizing film, electrical interference in EMG, or mechanical vibration in a force platform. Noise may be random or systematic, and different techniques must be used to eliminate different kinds of noise.

4.13 Smoothing

A class of techniques for reducing the effects of noise- For systematic noise, this usually involves a clear knowledge of the source of the noise (e.g., 60 Hz electrical interference). For attenuating the effects of random noise, a variety of techniques are used such as digital or electrical filtering, curve fitting, and averaging.

Synonym: Filtering and fitting of data (although these are actually smoothing techniques)

4.14 Cartesian Coordinate System

A system whereby a point can be located in space by three coordinates, usually denoted by (x, y, z), which express the perpendicular distance of the point along the respective axis from an origin. The three axes are mutually perpendicular.

The system is said to be right-handed if a rotation from x to y is clockwise and in the direction of positive z. A two-dimiensional Cartesian system involves mutually perpendicular x- and y-axes.

SECTION 5 MUSCLE MECHANICS

5.1 Contraction

In muscles, an active shortening of the muscle resulting in a reduction in the distance between the two ends of a muscle. It has, however, become popular to use the term to imply development of tension by a muscle whether or not shortening is underway. This usage is inexact and is not encouraged.

5.2 Muscle Action

The development of muscle tension (more appropriate than the term "contraction"). It can be applied to any type of tension development regardless of whether a muscle is lengthening, shortening, or maintaining the same length.

5.3 Eccentric Muscle Action

Muscle lengthening under tension. This lengthening occurs when the external force acting on the segment to which a muscle is attached causes a net moment that is greater than the moment that is being developed by the muscle and its synergists. Note: Use of the term "contraction" is clearly inappropriate for this type of muscle action.

5.4 Concentric Muscle Action

Muscle shortening under tension. This shortening occurs when the net moment developed by a muscle and its synergists is greater than the moment caused by the external forces acting on the segment to which the muscle is attached.

5.5 Isotonic Muscle Action

Muscle action that involves the production of a constant force. For in vivo muscle actions, the term is also commonly used both when the joint moment is constant over a range of motion and when a constant load is being moved through a distance. It is important to realize, however, that because of the leverage effects at the joint, the force developed by the muscles in both these cases will actually be changing, rendering them nonisotonic.

5.6 Isometric Muscle Action

Muscle action that involves no change in length of the muscle. This condition probably does not exist because the contractile components of a muscle shorten at the expense of the elastic structures in series even when the joint crossed by the muscle is fixed. The definition, therefore, is usually relaxed to mean the action of a muscle when no change exists in the distance between its points of attachment—referring to the joint and not to the muscle.

5.7 Isokinetic Muscle Action

Muscle action in which the rate of shortening or lengthening of the muscle is constant. Because joint geometry makes this impossible to determine in vivo, the definition is usually relaxed to apply either to a constant velocity of the load being lifted or resisted, or to a constant angular velocity of the joint.

Note: Both isokinetic and isotonic actions are fairly artificial when considered in the context of movements that occur in activities of daily living. Muscles usually shorten or lengthen at varying rates and with varying tensions. These actions are, nevertheless, useful for testing muscles under standardized conditions.

5.8 Origin

The source or beginning of a muscle. The term generally refers to the more fixed end or the more proximal end.

Note: This is an ambiguous term for any muscle that has attachments that are equally mobile or with both attachments in the same transverse plane. Use of the term tends to encourage the mistaken notion that muscles have their only action at the moveable rather than the fixed end. The same tension is, of course, applied to both ends. The term attachment is more appropriate for reference to either end of the muscle.

5.9 Insertion

The more distal attachment of the muscle or the attachment that is more mobile. Again, this is an ambiguous term for which attachment should be substituted (See Note in 5.8).

5.10 Muscular Efficiency

Expresses the ratio of the mechanical work done to the metabolic energy expanded (a widely used term in biomechanics and physiology). This definition has many problems, most of which are related to the definition of the work done. The major stumbling blocks to the establishment of a relationship are the storage of elastic energy in muscles, the different metabolic costs of positive and negative work, and the energy transfer between body segments.

5.11 "Spurt" and "Shunt" Muscles

A muscle's ability to exert rotatory force on a limb. This classification has, however, been challenged.[5] When the distal attachment is close to the joint at which the muscle acts, the muscle is called a spurt muscle. This is said to result in a greater rotatory component compared with its stabilizing component. The shunt muscles have their more proximal attachment close to the joint, and their action is said to be more for stabilization than for rotation. The biceps brachii muscle is often presented as an example of a spurt muscle and the brachioradialis muscle as an example of a shunt muscle.

5.12 Tension-Length Relationship

The variation in force output of a muscle, with the same neural input, over a range of lengths. The reasons for this variation include a change in the number of possible active sites for cross-bridge formation and the effect of the elastic tissues that are in parallel with the contractile tissue. A typical tension-length curve for human muscle is shown in Figure 12.

Note: The moment that the muscle can develop about a joint will vary both according to the tension-length relationship and as a function of the geometry of the joint (the location of its attachments and so forth). A typical joint angle-maximum moment curves shown in Figure 13.

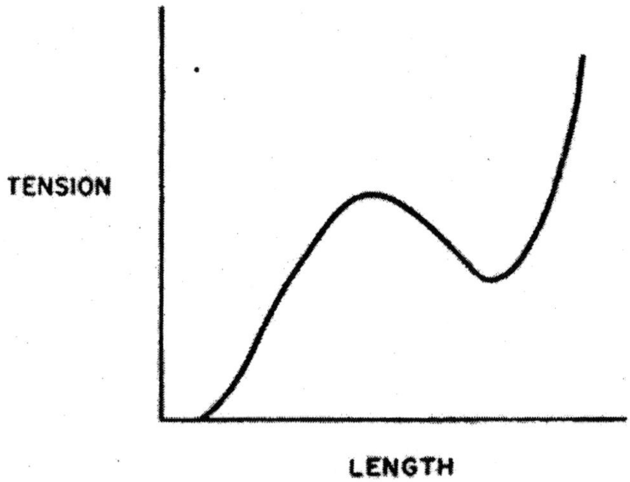

Figure 12. Typical tension-length curve for an intact human muscle. This curve includes both active and passive components.

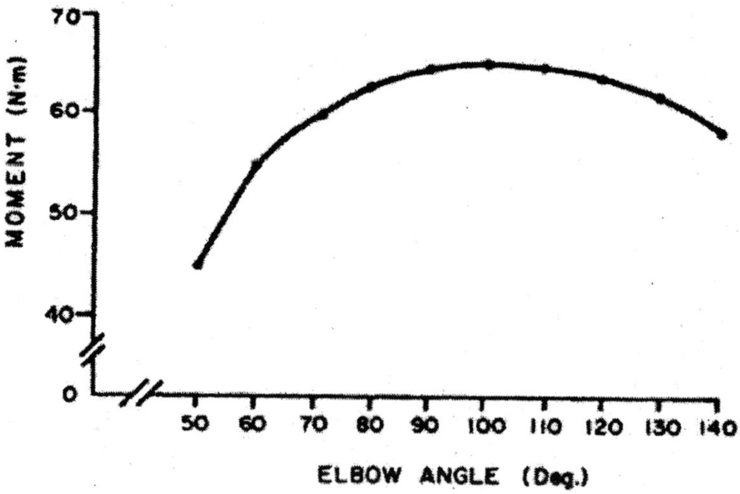

Figure 13. Illustration of joint angle-maximum moment curve for elbow flexion.

5.13 Force-Velocity relationship

At any given length, the speed of shortening or lengthening of a muscle that is stimulated at a constant level will depend on the force that is applied to the ends of the muscle. The Hill equation, best known of the force-velocity equations, describes mathematically the fact that light loads can be lifted quickly but heavy loads only slowly.[6] Although it is often stated that maximal muscle force is available at zero velocity (isometric action), the highest loads are achieved during eccentric muscle action.

5.14 Muscle Model

Any mechanical or mathematical model that describes the function of muscle tissue during activity and rest. The best known of these is the three-component Hill[6] model that postulates a contractile element, a series elastic element, and a parallel elastic element in the configuration seen in Figure 14.

MECHANICS OF MATERIALS

6.1 Density

The mass of matter in a given space, that is, the mass per unit volume.

Note:	Pure water at 0° C has a density of 1.0. Objects with a density greater than 1 will sink in water; those with a density less than 1 will float in water.
Units:	SI—kilogram per cubic meter (kg/m^3)
	US Customary—pound per cubic foot (lb/ft^3)
Symbol:	ρ

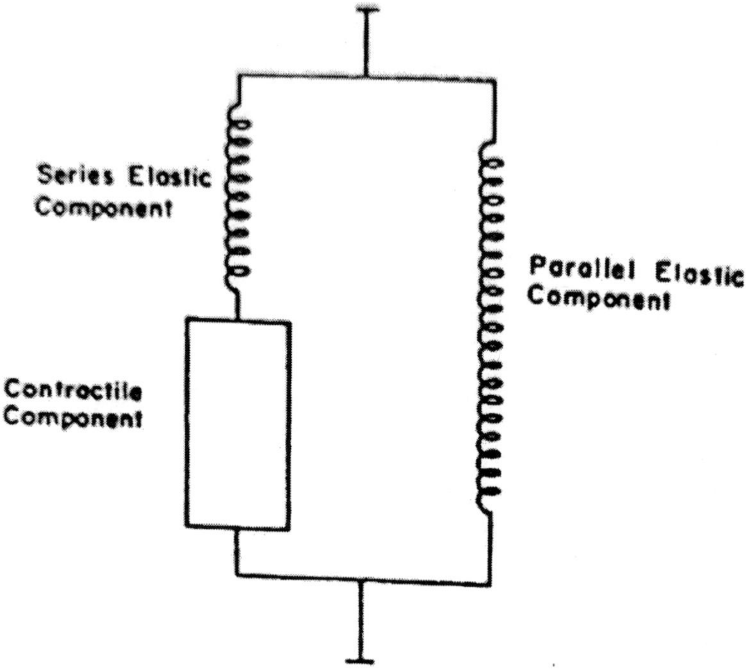

Figure 14. Three-component Hill model of muscle.

6.2 Tension

A loading mode in which collinear forces acting in opposite directions tend to pull an object apart. In general, a tensile force will cause the length of the body to be increased and the width to be narrowed.

6.3 Distraction

The movement of two surfaces away from each other. In joints, distraction refers to a form of dislocation where the two joint surfaces are separated but retain their ligamentous integrity.

6.4 Compression

A loading mode in which collinear forces are acting in opposite directions to push the material together. Compression usually results in a shortening and widening of the material.

6.5 Stress

Force per unit area that develops within a structure in response to externally applied loads. The stress may be tensile or compressive depending on the mode of loading. The stress may also be normal (changing the length in a structure) or shear (changing the angle in a structure).

Units:	SI—Pascal (Pa) US Customary—pound force per square inch (psi)
Synonym:	pressure but not strain
Symbol:	σ

6.6 Strain

Deformation that occurs at a point in a structure under loading. Two basic types of strain exist: normal strain, which is a change in length, and shear strain, which is a change in angle. Normal strain is the ratio of deformation (lengthening or shortening) to original length. Shear strain is the amount of angular deformation that occurs in a structure. For example, a rectangle drawn on one face of a solid before a shear stress is applied will appear as a parallelogram during the application of a shear stress.

Units:	Because it is a ratio, strain is dimensionless but it is often expressed as percent strain (i.e., the above definition multiplied by 100). Because rigid materials deform by only small amounts, the "pseudo units" of microstrains are often used. One microstrain represents a deformation of one ten-thousandth of 1 percent.
Synonym:	elongation
Symbol:	ε

6.7 Modulus of Elasticity

The ratio of stress to strain at any point in the elastic region of deformation, yielding a value for stiffness. The stiffer the material, the higher the modulus. The moduli in compression and tension are different for most biological materials because they are anisotropic (See 6.13).

Synonym: Young's modulus, modulus, elastic modulus

Units: Because it is the ratio of stress to strain and strain is dimensionless (See 9.4), modulus of elasticity has the units of stress.

SI—Pascal (Pa) or more often newtons per square centimeter (N/cm^2)

US Customary—pounds per square inch (psi) .

Note on Units: Some typical values of the modulus of elasticity are bone: approx. 5 GPa (wet human femur in compression) and steel: approx. 20 GPa.

Symbol: E

6.8 Elastic Deformation

A strain in a material that is entirely reversible when the stress is released.

6.9 Plastic Deformation

A strain in a material that is permanent and will not recover when the stress is released

6.10 Strain Rate

The speed at which a strain-producing load is applied or the first derivative of strain.

Note: When data on the mechanical properties of biological tissue are presented, it is important to state the strain rate at which the data were collected. Because most tissue is viscoelastic (see 6.19) the properties will be rate dependent. Most testing machines that stress tissue samples are unable to achieve strain rates that are biologically realistic. All published values on biological materials must be viewed with this limitation in mind.

Units: SI—meter/sec (m/s) or original lengths/sec

US Customary—inches per second (in/sec) (in/s)

6.11 Strain Energy

The energy that a material can absorb as a result of the change of shape resulting from applied stress. The work done, stored as strain energy in the material, is the product of the average force (½P) and the deformation.

$$U = \tfrac{1}{2}\,(P^2 \cdot L)/A \cdot E \qquad (18)$$

where L = material length, A = material area, and E = modulus of elasticity. Graphically, the area under a load-deformation curve represents the strain energy stored in the material during the application of stress.

Units: SI—newton meters (N · m)

US Customary—foot pound force (ft · lbf)

Synonym: energy stored

Symbol: U

6.12 Isotropic

A material that has no directional structure and exhibits the same mechanical properties when loaded in different directions. For example, in an isotropic material (e.g., a sheet of natural rubber), the elastic properties are identical in all directions.

6.13 Anisotropic

A material that has a directional structure and exhibits different mechanical properties when loaded in different directions. For example, because the structure of bone or tendon is different in the transverse and the longitudinal directions, the modulus of elasticity varies according to the direction in which the load is imposed.

6.14 Bending

The result of applying a load to a structure such that it bends about an axis. The structure will be experiencing a combination of tension and compression on opposite surfaces.

6.15 Neutral Axis

The central plane in which the tensile and compressive stresses and strains resulting from bending equal zero.

6.16 Bending Moment

A quantitative measure of the tendency of a force to bend a structure. It is calculated as the product of the applied force and the perpendicular distance from the point of force application to the axis.

Units: SI—newton meters (N · m)

US Customary—foot pound force (ft · lbf)

6.17 Bone Remodeling

The ability of the bone to adapt, by changing its size, shape, and structure, to the mechanical demands placed on it. The idea that living bone can functionally adapt to internal stresses and strains was first advanced by Julius Wolff in 1884. Wolff's law states that bone is laid down where needed and resorbed where not needed. The remodeling may be either external (a change in the external shape of the bone) or internal (a change in the porosity, mineral content, and density of bone).

6.18 Fatigue

The failure of a material caused by loading.

6.19 Viscoelasticity

The behavior of materials that exhibit the features of hysteresis (See 6.20) stress relaxation (See 6.21) and creep (See 6.22).

Note: Modeling of viscoelastic behavior must include elements such as dashpots (fluid-filled damping units) that can absorb energy, whereas elastic behavior can be satisfactorily modeled by perfect springs, which return all the energy they store.

6.20 Hysteresis

A phenomenon in which a body, when subjected to cyclic loading, exhibits a stress-strain relationship during the loading process different from that in the unloading process (Fig. 15).

Note: When a stress-strain diagram for the cyclic loading of a material that shows hysteresis is drawn, the result is sometimes called a hysteresis loop. The maximum width of the loop (along the strain axis) divided by the largest value for strain expressed in percent is called the hysteresis.

Units: percent %

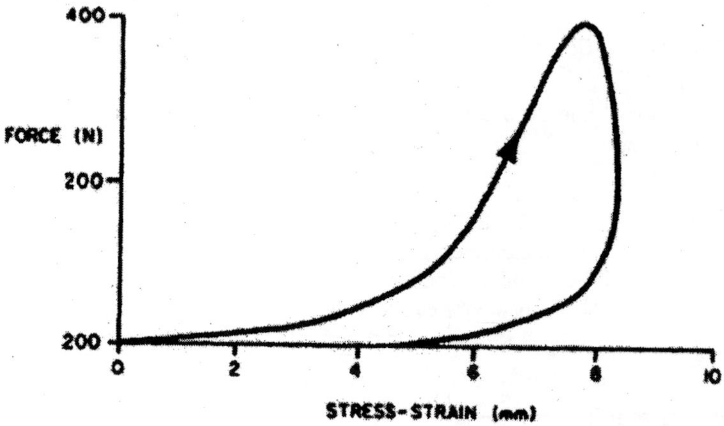

Figure 15. Hysteresis loop for the tissue of the heel pad.

6.21 Stress Relaxation

The phenomenon in which the stress in a sample, which was suddenly strained and then maintained at the final strain, gradually decreases with time.

6.22 Creep

Progressive deformation of soft tissues because of constant loading over an extended period of time. This is typically demonstrated by suddenly stressing a sample and then holding the load constant afterwards. If the sample continues to deform, then it is said to be exhibiting creep.

6.23 Shock Absorption

The progressive damping of an applied force. Damping is a complex, generally nonlinear, phenomenon that exists whenever energy is dissipated.

Note: It is important to realize that force cannot be absorbed. A shock absorbent material acts to change the momentum of an impact over a longer period of time than a nonshock absorbent material.

Instrumentation

7.1 Transducer

A measuring device that converts one form of energy into another. An electrical displacement transducer, for example, converts kinetic energy from movement into electrical energy.

Synonym: sensor

7.2 Force Platform

An electromechanical device that gives electrical signals proportional to the components of force acting on it. The most common use of a force platform is to measure the reaction forces and center of pressure between the foot and the floor during locomotor activities. The resultant force is usually resolved into three orthogonal components (See 4.14). Force transducers used in a force platform are usually either strain gauges, which change their electrical resistance with strain or piezoelectric elements, which generate charge when stressed.

Synonym: force plate but not pressure plate (because no estimate of contact area is usually available to compute stress)

7.3 Pressure Platform

A device that consists of a matrix of elements that are small force transducers of known area. If this area is sufficiently small, the force on each element can be considered uniformly distributed and, thus, an estimate of pressure is available.

Note: This device gives more information concerning load distribution than a force platform because the pressures acting on various anatomical regions can be measured rather than just the resultant force acting on, for example, the whole foot.

7.4 Accelerometer

A transducer that measures acceleration. It usually consists of an inertial mass that exerts a forces against an element, such as a beam, whose resulting strain is then measured.

Note: Like force, acceleration cannot be directly measured and must be estimated from the effects of a force. A major problem associated with making acceleration measurements on body segments is that the transducer is generally fixed to soft tissues rather than bone. The directional effect of the transducer is also a problem because it is always under the influence of gravity.

7.5 Cyclograph

A device used in the collection of kinematic data. It consists of a disk with a sector that is rotated in front of a camera with an open shutter. The subject moves in front of a black background and an image is registered on the film of the posture of the body each time the sector is opposite the camera lens. The result, with multiple images on a single piece of film, is similar to a stroboscopic picture.

7.6 Stroboscopy

Multiple image photography in which the camera shutter is held open for a time exposure, and strobe lighting is used to illuminate the subject at designated intervals. Another approach is to affix tiny lights to important body landmarks and flash them at a predetermined rate.

The disadvantages of the technique are that the movement must be performed in the dark, and that if a limb segment moves through the same space on more than one occasion, the result is difficult to interpret.

7.7 High-Speed Cinematography

The most frequently used method of examining human motion. Film is taken at a higher rate than the usual 24 frames per second (fps) and subsequently analyzed frame-by-frame using a digitizer. Traditionally, analyses yielding only the two-dimensional coordinates of body landmarks in a single plane have been performed (See 7.6). Biomechanical studies generally use cameras capable of 500 fps or less although frame rates greater than 5,000,000 fps are possible. Synonym: slow-motion cinematography

7.8 Three-Dimensional Cinematography

A technique in which generally two or more motion picture cameras are used to obtain spatial coordinates of landmarks on the body in three dimensions (x, y, z). A variety of techniques is used, but all of them involve extensive analysis and computation.

Synonym: 3D cine

7.9 Digitizer

A device that is capable of acquiring planar coordinates in numerical form. In biomechanics, the most frequent use of a digitizer is to convert the location of body markers on the projected image of a film into numbers that can be processed by a computer.

Synonym: graphics tablet, digitizing tablet or table

7.10 ELGON

A potentiometer (variable resistor) that is attached to the body to measure a joint angle. The axis of the potentiometer is aligned with the joint axis and the device gives an output voltage that is proportional to joint angle.

Note: Most potentiometers assume there is a single fixed axis of rotation for the joint—an assumption that is not generally true. Other problems with electrogoniometry include fixation of the device to the body and possible alteration of the movement because of the attachment.

Synonym: The acronym stands for electrogoniometer.

7.11 Optoelectronic Methods

A new generation of devices for measuring the displacement of body landmarks using optical and electronic methods to produce an immediate or on-line estimate.

Note: Because cinematography is such a laborious process, these methods offer considerable promise, particularly for motion analysis in a clinical environment where turn-around time is important. At present, however, most of these methods cannot approach the accuracy of cinematography.

7.12 Selspot

An optoelectronic technique for measuring displacement in which light from a pulsing infrared light target attached to the body is focused onto a special diode inside a camera. The output from the diode, after suitable processing, yields an estimate of the ordinates of the target. Many such targets can be placed on the body and their locations estimated in rapid sequence.

7.13 POLGON

An optoelectronic device for measuring angular displacement that is composed of an optical projector and a number of receivers attached to the body parts under investigation. The light emitted from the projector is directed at the subject through a rotating polaroid screen. Joint angles are available on-line as functions of time.

Synonym: The acronym stands for polarized light goniometer.

7.14 Microcomputer

A computer that has the major arithmetic and logical functions all on one integrated chip called a microprocessor. This chip is the heart of the system around which the various other parts of the computer are arranged. Each major type of microprocessor chip has its own number that identifies both the set of instructions it recognizes and its word length. The Apple II, for example, is built around the 6502 microprocessor chip, and the IBM PC is based on the 68000.

Note: Many new devices that are seen in the clinic or laboratory are now "microprocessor controlled," which means they contain a small dedicated microprocessor with preset instructions that respond to input from the control panel or external inputs.

Synonym: microprocessor

7.15 Minicomputer

A computer that is built on a larger scale than a microcomputer so that its processing functions are distributed among several main units. A minicomputer is typically found in a laboratory or clinical environment where it can respond to the needs of a number of users simultaneously. It usually has a variety of peripheral devices for storage and output (e.g., disk and tape drives, and line printers), and a fairly complex operating system (see 7.16).

7.16 Hardware

The actual machines used in data collection and processing as distinct from the programs or instructions that cause them to operate in a given manner.

7.17 Software

Sets of instructions called programs that cause a computer to execute certain operations. These instructions may be written in a high-level language like BASIC, PASCAL, or FORTRAN, or in a lower-level language such as Assembly Language (the higher the level, the closer to the English language). Some categories of software follow:

1. User programs—programs written by individual users.
2. System programs—programs that control the housekeeping functions of the computer—such as input/output and deciding which user to respond to at a given time. Such programs are often stored in ROM (See 7.18).
3. Application programs—programs that are sold to perform a certain function—perhaps statistics or patient record keeping. Sometimes called canned programs.
4. Word processors—programs that work with words rather than numbers as their basic elements. They allow easy editing of text and the generation of form letters with different inserts.

7.18 Read Only Memory (ROM)

An area of computer memory where programs supplied by the manufacturer are stored semipermanently. This form of memory cannot be overwritten by a user.

Synonym: The acronym stands for read only memory.

7.19 Random Access Memory (RAM)

An area of computer memory that is available for user programs, data, and other temporary uses. It can be overwritten continually.

Synonym: The acronym stands for random access memory.

7.20 On-Line

A term used for data that can be processed and displayed immediately after collection. The opposite term, off-line, implies a lag between data collection and the availability of the results. On-line data collection and analysis are clearly important in a clinical context where feedback is to be given either to the patient or to those who are treating the patient.

SECTION 8 BODY SEGMENT VARIABLES

8.1 Anthropometry

A branch of biomechanics that deals with the measurement of the dimensions, mass, and mass distribution of the human body and its segments.

8.2 Link System

An assumption underlying most anthropometric models of the body that states the body is composed of a system of rigid links whose ends are connected by smooth pin joints. Pheasant has contrasted the use of this assumption with the analogy that a human limb segment is better characterized as "a series of fluid filled sacks loosely connected to a set of deformable rods."[7] To cope with such a characterization in biomechanical calculations of body movement would render most problems insoluble.

8.3 Body Segment Factors

Estimates of the lengths, masses, location of the centers of mass, and moments of inertia of body segments that are required for biomechanical analysis of human motion.

8.4 Cadaveric Techniques

The segmentation and measurement of cadavers to determine body segment variables. The value of dissection studies lies in their potential for providing a basis for prediction of segmental variables in living subjects. For example, cadaver studies have shown that the mass of the thigh is approximately 10 percent of total body mass. The scope of inference is, however, limited both by the nature of the samples (less than 50 cadavers have been studied and most were geriatric Caucasian males) and by the assumption that cadaver data can be applied to living subjects.

8.5 Mathematical Models

The modeling of segments of the body by geometrical shapes as a method of predicting body segment variables. Segments are usually assumed to be homogeneous right or elliptical cylinders, spheres, ellipsoids of revolution, or frustra of cones. The advantage of these models is that estimates are available for all variables; the major disadvantage is that of oversimplification.

8.6 Regression Equation Techniques

The use of multiple correlation and regression techniques to improve on the prediction of body segment variables from cadaveric data. This generally yields an equation for segmental mass, for example, where factors other than (or in addition to) total body mass are included as predictors. In the best known example of this technique, three equations are available for each variable, each using successively more predictors and resulting in an improved standard error of the estimate.[8]

SECTION 9 UNITS

9.1 Background to Systems of Units

All units systems have in common the fact that units for the three fundamental quantities of mass, length, and time are defined arbitrarily to give what are sometimes called the base units. The units of all other quantities are expressed in terms of these base units to form what are called derived units.

The set of units that is still in current use in everyday life in the United States is the British system based on the pound, the foot, and the second. These units have long been out of favor with the scientific community and have even been abandoned by the British for everyday and scientific use. They have therefore been referred to in this paper by the more appropriate title as US Customary units. The generally accepted system of scientific units is the Systeme International d'Unites (the International System or SI system) that was agreed on in 1960.[9,10] The system is based on the kilogram, the meter, and the second. This system is the only one now accepted by most scientific journals and should always be used. Conversion factors between the SI and British units are presented in Section 9.5.

Each unit has a standard abbreviation and care should be taken to use both the correct letter(s) and the correct case (upper or lower). When the units for a derived quantity are written (e.g., those compound units formed by multiplication), the abbreviations for the elementary quantities should be written with the product dot separating them (e.g., N · m for newton meter).

When the size of a quantity becomes very large or small, it is customary to use powers of 10 (positive or negative) to make the number before the multiplier between 1 and 10 or to use standard prefixes that imply a given multiple of powers of 10. Examples of this would be as follows:

5.32×10^3 N or 5.32 kN rather than 5320 N (19)

7.13×10^{-4} sec or 0.713 msec rather than .000713 sec (20)

Notice that no space exists between the prefix and the symbol for the unit. The most common of the standard series of prefixes that should be used with their correct abbreviation are listed below. They progress by multiples of 1,000.

Unit Prefixes and Abbreviations		
Prefix	**Abbreviation**	**Multiply By**
Giga	G	1,000,000,000
Mega	M	1,000,000
Kilo	k	1,000
Centi	c	1/100
Milli	m	1/1,000
Micro	μ	1/1,000,000

9.2 Definitions of the Base Units

Mass: The kilogram is a unit of mass and not force. The basis of this unit is the mass of a physical specimen—The International Prototype Kilo gram—kept in Paris. A replica of this physical specimen is kept at the National Bureau of Standards, Washington, DC.

Length: The SI unit of length is the meter. This was originally defined at the time of the French Revolution as 1 /10,000,000 of the distance between the North Pole and the Equator. Despite the primitive methods of making measurements available at the time, they made a remarkably close approximation. Recently the definition has been standardized using the wavelength of an emission from an isoe of krypton.

Time: The original definition of the second was 1/86,400th of the mean solar day. The modern definition is, like that of length, based on the atomic properties of a radioactive element, in this case, cesium 133.

9.3 Derived Units

Force: Using Newton's second law, the SI unit of force, the newton (N), is defined as that force that gives a mass of 1 kg an acceleration of 1 m per second per second.

Note: The confusion in the English system between the pound as a unit of mass and the pound force as a unit of force is not present in the SI system. The pound force (lbf) is defined as the force under a 1-pound mass when it is stationary on a surface in the earth's gravitational field. For obvious reasons, the pound force is called a gravitational unit because its definition using Newton's law can be stated as

$$1 \text{ force unit} = 1 \text{ mass unit} \cdot g \quad (21)$$

In the definition of absolute units (such as the newton), Newton's second law has the form

1 force unit = 1 mass unit · 1 acceleration unit (22)

Neither the pound force nor the analogous metric unit—the kilogram force—should be used.

Pressure: The SI unit of pressure is the Pascal (Pa). This is the pressure experienced when a force of 1 newton (N) is distributed over an area of 1-square meter (m^2). This unit defines an amount of pressure that is extremely small for most biomechanical studies of gross body movement. For example, the average pressure underneath a size nine foot when a 75-kg (165-lb) person is standing on one leg is approximately 70,000 Pa. Thus, the units of kilopascals (kPa) and megapascals (mPa) are frequently used.

Work: When a force of 1 newton moves through a distance of 1 meter, 1 joule (J) of work is said to have been done.

Energy: Same units as work.

Power: When 1 joule of work is done in a period of 1 second (set), the power output is said to be 1 watt (W).

Moment: The units for moment or torque are newton meters (N · m), that is a force of 1 newton applied at a distance of 1 meter from an axis produces a turning moment or torque of 1 newton meter. This unit must not be simplified to joules because the joule is not a unit of moment.

Plane Angle: One radian is the angle subtended between two lines joining the center of a circle with two points on the circumference that are the radius of the circle apart. This unit is dimensionless.

9.4 Dimensions

When manipulating quantities with a variety of units (e.g., in equations of motion), the concepts of dimensions and dimensional analysis are frequently useful.[10] In this approach, quantities are manipulated as combinations of the "base" quantities of mass, length, and time, from which, as stated earlier, most other "derived quantities" can be obtained. The symbols of dimensional analysis are [M], [L], and [T], and units are ignored in favor of these quantities. For example, the derived quantity of force is obtained from the product of mass and acceleration. Acceleration is itself a derived quantity that has dimensions of $[L][T]^{-2}$. It may help to think of the units that are meters (length) per second (time) per second (time). Thus, the final dimensions of force are $[M][L][T]^{-2}$.

Dimensional analysis can be extremely useful in finding errors in equations. For example, in calculating the moment of a force about a point, the dimensions of the answer, which is calculated as force multiplied by a distance, will be $[M][L]^2[T]^{-2}$. Suppose, in the calculation of a moment equation, the following result were obtained:

$$F_x \cdot x \cdot \cos\theta + F_y \cdot \cos\theta = M \quad (23)$$

where F_x and F_y are force components, x is a distance, θ is an angle, and M is a moment.

Dimensional analysis would reveal the following:

$$[M][L][T]^{-2}[L] + [M][L][T]^{-2} = [M][L]^2[T]^{-2} \quad (24)$$

The equations are said to be "dimensionally inhomogeneous" because all additive terns do not have the same dimensions. Inspection reveals that the distance component in the second term was missed out and when this error is corrected, all terms will. have the same dimensions.

9.5 Conversion Factors

Mass 1 kg = 2.240 lb

	1 lb = 0.453 kg
Length	1 m = 1.094 yd
	1 m = 3.281 ft
	1 m = 39.370 in
	1 yd = 0.914 m
	1 ft = 0.305 m
	1 in = 0.0254 m
Force	1 N = 0.225 lbf
	1 lbf = 4.448 N
	1 kgf = 9.81 N
Pressure	1 kPa = 0.145 psi
	1 bar = 100 kPa
	1 atm = 101.3 kPa
Work/Energy	1 J = 0.737 ft · lbf
	1 J = 0.243 calories
	1 ft· lbf = 1.356 J
Power	1 W = 0.737 ft· lbf/sec
	1 ft· lbf/sec = 1.356 W
	1 hp = 746 W

Moment	1 N· m = 0.737 ft · lbf
	1 ft· lbf/sec = 1.356 N · m
Angle	1 radian = 57.3°
	1° = 0.0174 radians
	radians = 180°
	60 minutes of arc = 1°
	60 seconds of arc = 1 minute of arc

Principles of Biomechanics

Basic Biomechanics

To understand control of the musculoskeletal system we must study *kinetics*, not just kinematics.

Kinetics = kinematics (study of motion) + dynamics (study of forces)

Kinematics	= Study of Motion
Dynamics	= Study of Forces (causing motion)
Kinetics	= Kinematics + Dynamics
Statics	= Kinetics with forces in equilibrium

- Statics analyses kinetics with forces and moments in equilibrium ($\Sigma F = 0$, $\Sigma M = 0$).
  - Applies to bodies at rest or uniform motion (constant velocity i.e., no accelerations)
  - Newton's Laws 1 and 2

- Muscles generate force which is translated into a joint moment.
    - Muscles generate moments not necessarily movements

- Moments (torques) = Force x moment arm (d)
    - Moment arm = distance from axis of rotation to the line of action of the force, and perpendicular to it.

Statics analyses kinetics with forces and moments in equilibrium

(I.e. sum of F = 0, sum of M = 0).

Applies to bodies at rest **or in uniform motion** (constant velocity i.e., no accelerations)

Muscles generate force which is translated into a joint moment.

Remember:

Muscles generate moments, not necessarily movements

Moments (torques) = Force x moment arm (d)

Moment arm = perpendicular distance from axis of rotation to the *line of action* of the force.

Functional Anatomy

Tissue Mechanics

1. General Concepts of Tissue Mechanics

- Functional basis for understanding resistance to fracture

    - Mechanical Properties of Solids

    Properties of Ligaments (Week 2)
    Properties of Bone

2. Factors affecting mechanical properties

- material properties
- Structural properties
- anisotropy
- Bone microstructure

3. Viscoelasticity

- Viscoelasticity of biomaterials

4. Assessment of Bone fragility in vivo

- In vivo strain analysis
- Bone densitometry

Elastic Properties of Solids:

When we pull on any tissue (bone, tendons and skin) it will stretch. The stiffness of the material is defined as

Stiffness = Force Change / Change in Length = $\Delta F/\Delta l$

Bone is stiffer than skin because it requires much more force to stretch bone in the same amount as skin. However, what about a thick bone and a thin one? Or what about a single rubber band and a bunch of 10 bands? It takes 10 times as much force to stretch the 10 bands compared to the single one. With the equation above, we have identified the stiffness of a structure, not the stiffness of the material that the structure is made of.

To determine and compare the stiffness of materials, we have to normalise for the size of the structure.

Force is normalised for the cross-sectional area of the structure, and change in length is normalised for the original length of the structure:

Stress = Force/Cross Section = $\sigma = F/A$

Strain = Change in Length / Original Length = $\varepsilon = \Delta l/lo$

Thus we can define normalised stiffness as:

Normalised Stiffness or Young's Modulus = $E = \Delta\sigma/\varepsilon$

Young's modulus is often referred to as the elastic modulus.

Hooke's law states that the elongation (or strain) of material is proportionally related to the amount of force (or stress). In other words, stiffness and Young's modulus are constant an independent of the applied force.

The equation above can be rewritten to predict the stress as a function of strain:

$\Delta\sigma = E^*\varepsilon$ and ΔF = Stiffness * Δl

Viscous properties of fluids

Fluids behave in a similar way as solids, with one major difference: the force (stress) generated in a fluid does not depend on elongation (see last equation above) but on the speed of length change. In formula:

$\Delta\sigma = \eta^* d\varepsilon/dt$ and ΔF = Viscosity * dl/dt = Viscosity * velocity

The symbol η is the normalised viscosity (compare with E). The viscosity property is a bit harder to visualise then elasticity. Think of a tank filled with water and you move your hand through it (or you are swimming in a pool).

You feel resistance against the movement as long as you are moving! That is, the resistance depends on movement per se, or better on the speed of movement (the faster you try to move the more resistance you experience).

As soon as you stop moving, no matter where your hand is in the tank, the resistance stops. Thus, the resistance (force, stress) does not depend on the amount of movement (hand position).

Furthermore, the direction of the movement does not play a role, in contrast to elasticity of solids.

Just for a moment, replace the water in the tank by a spring attached to one of the walls. Now, the hand force depends on the amount of movement not on the speed.

Example: Normalised Load-Deformation Curve

(Stress-Strain Curve)

Specimen Characteristics

Specimen	Area (m^2)	Lo (m)	Lult (m)	Force (N)	Stress (Pa)	Strain (%)
1	0.2	0.5	1.0	10	50	100
2	0.4	0.5	1.0	20	50	100

Note that specimen 2 is the same length, but has twice the cross-sectional area

Stiffness vs Elastic Modulus

Stiffness			
Stiffness 1 =	$\Delta F / \Delta L$	Stiffness 2 =	$\Delta F / \Delta L$
=	10 / 0.5	=	20 / 0.5
=	20 N/m	=	40 N/m
Elastic Modulus			
E 1 =	$\Delta \delta / \varepsilon$	E2 =	$\Delta \delta / \varepsilon$
=	50 /1	=	50 / 1
=	50 Pa	=	50 Pa

Specimen 2 turns out to have twice the stiffness of specimen 1 because of its greater size (structural property), but when normalized for differences in geometry has the same elastic modulus (material property).

Fundamental Biomechanical Concepts

Kinematics (Direction, Extent, Speed of Motion)

TRANSLATORY Movement (typical units)	**ROTATORY Movement (typical units)**
DISPLACEMENT / DISTANCE (in.; cm)	ANGULAR DISPLACEMENT (degrees)
VELOCITY (in/sec ; cm/sec)	ANGULAR VELOCITY (deg/sec)
ACCELERATION (in/sec/sec)	ANGULAR ACCELERATION (deg/sec/sec)

Kinematics of the knee during gait

The first graph illustrates the knee's angular displacement (in degrees) during the gait cycle. The second and third graphs demonstrate angular velocity (in degrees/sec) and angular acceleration (in degrees/sec/sec), respectively.

The graphs also illustrate how angular velocity, the rate of change in joint angle, reflects the instantaneous slope of the displacement curve. Likewise, angular acceleration, the rate of change in angular velocity, represents the instantaneous slope of the velocity curve.

Knee movement during the gait cycle

The knee:

- Flexes during loading response (0 to 10 percent)
- Extends during midstance and most of terminal stance (10 to 50%)
- Flexes degrees during preswing and initial swing (50 to 70%)

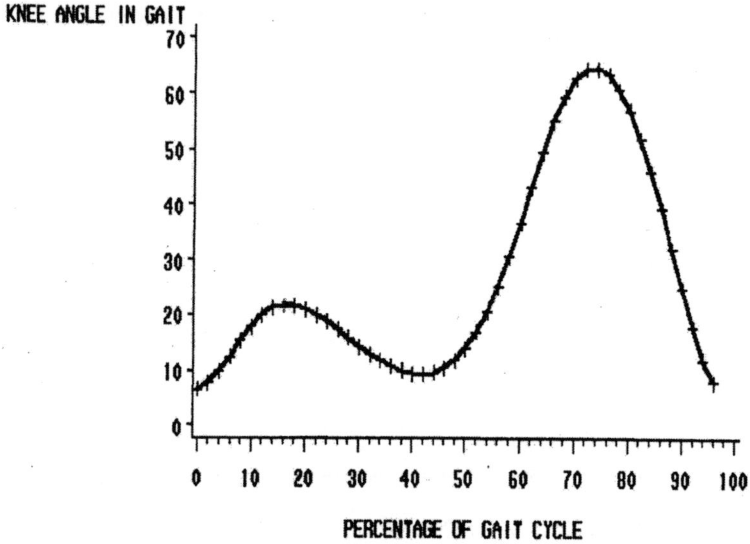

Knee flexion during loading response
(0 to 10 percent of gait cycle)

- In this closed kinematic chain, the screw-home mechanism reverses:
  - Femur glides anteriorly on tibia
  - Anterior femoral glide begins earlier on medial condyles, causing external femoral rotation
- Tibia also internally rotates
  - Tibial rotation imparted by pelvic rotation
  - Tibial rotation produces subtalar pronation

Knee Extension during Midstance

- In this closed kinematic chain, the knee exhibits the "screw-home" mechanism of terminal rotation:
  - Femur glides posteriorly on tibia
  - Posterior femoral glide persists on medial condyles because of the length of their articular surfaces, causing internal femoral rotation
- Tibia also rotates externally

- Tibial rotation imparted by pelvic rotation
- Tibial rotation produces subtalar supination

Kinetics

- Definitions of kinetic terms
- Static and dynamic equilibrium of forces and moments
- Equations of motion
- Effect of a force on a joint surface
    - effect of a gravitational force on the hip joint
    - effect of a muscle force on the hip joint

Kinetics: terms defined

The familiar formulas for translational ("straight-line") motion have analogous equations for rotational motion (motion around a joint axis.)

	for TRANSLATIONAL MOTION	for ROTATIONAL MOTION
FORCE (F)	F=ma (measured in lbs or Newtons)	M=I*g (measured in ft*lbs or N*m) called MOMENT OF FORCE MOMENT TORQUE note: I=MOMENT OF INERTIA g=ANGULAR ACCELERATION
WORK (W)	W=Fd	W=Mr r=angular displacement (in radians, which are "dimensionless")
ENERGY	E=Fd	E=Mr

(E)		
POWER (P)	P=dE/dt P=F(ds/dt)	P=dE/dt P=M(dr/dt) P=Mw where M=joint moment w=angular velocity

Equilibrium of forces and moments

When one force acts on mass, we can apply Newton's Law:

F=ma

When several forces act on a mass, we simply sum their individual effects on the mass:

$$F_1 + F_2 + F_3 + F_4 + \dots F_n = ma$$

Thus,

$$\sum_i F_i = m\,a$$

Similarly, we can analyze the effects of several moments of force around an axis of movement:

$$\sum_i M_i = I\,\ddot{\theta}$$

Where the total moment equals the product of I, the segment's moment of inertia around an axis of movement, and its angular acceleration around that axis.

Static equilibrium

We refer to a situation as static when a mass' acceleration (j in the equation above), either in a straight line or around a joint axis, is equal to zero, or very nearly zero. Acceleration is zero when the mass is at rest, that is, not moving or moving at a constant velocity.

In this case, the equation that defines static equilibrium is:

EM=0

and the sum of the moments acting around a joint axis is zero. For example, in this frontal plane view of the lower extremity,

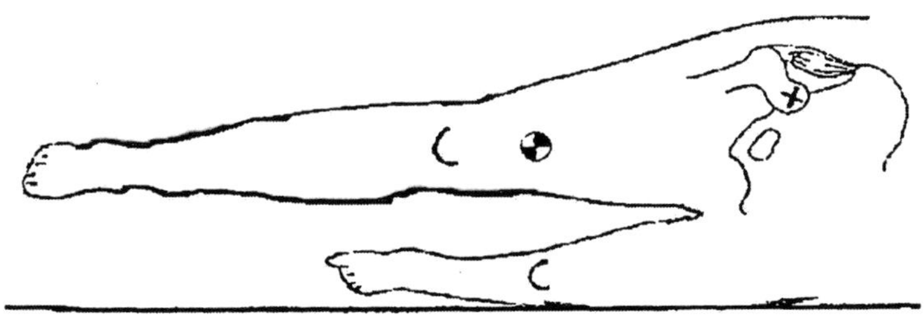

the sum of moments producing hip adduction are perfectly balanced by moments that produce hip abduction.

Thus,

$$M_m = M_g$$

$$F_g s_g = F_m s_m$$

$$F_m = (F_g s_g)/s_m$$

Dynamic Equilibrium

We often treat movement problems as if they are static, assuming that accelerations are nearly zero. These assumptions make movement problems easy to solve. When these simplifying assumptions are unwarranted, when a joint does not move at a constant velocity (including v=0) and an angular acceleration equal to zero, we must deal with the more complex equilibrium equation:

EM=Ij

where the total moment that acts on the joint (EM, the sum of individual moments) is measurable and nonzero.

Total moment = **(internal) joint moment**
- gravity moment
- interaction moments

The joint moment is calculated as a residual once the other moments are known:

Joint moment = **Total joint moment**
+ gravity moment
+ interaction moments

Where

- Total moment is the product of the joint angular acceleration and the segment's moment of inertia about the joint.
- Gravity moment is that produced by gravity acting on the segment center of mass
- Interaction moments or torques include those produced by inertial, centripetal, and coriolis forces.

Equations of motion

The equations of motion permit us to model movements mathematically. One of the most useful equations comes from Newton's second law of motion, which states that the sum of all forces acting on an object is equal to the product of the object's mass and its rate of change of velocity, or acceleration.

$$\sum_i F_i = m\,a$$

An analogous equation for rotational movement relates the sum of moments acting on an object to the product of that object's moment of inertia around an axis of rotation and its angular acceleration.

$$\sum_i M_i = I\,\ddot{\theta}$$

The sum of moments, symbolized by the left side of this equation, is composed of a variety of individual moments, including

- ground reaction moments
- gravity and inertial moments
- joint moments, produced by forces in muscle and other soft tissue

Because many movements combine straight-line translational movement with rotation around some axis, we often must employ both equations.

Gravity's (body weight's) effect on the hip joint surface during unilateral stance

Using the technique of vector resolution, we can analyze the effects that gravitational forces have on the hip's articular surfaces.

We begin by drawing a red, dashed reference line that approximates the hip joint surface's orientation. The surface is curved, so we estimate the orientation of a line that is tangent to that curve.

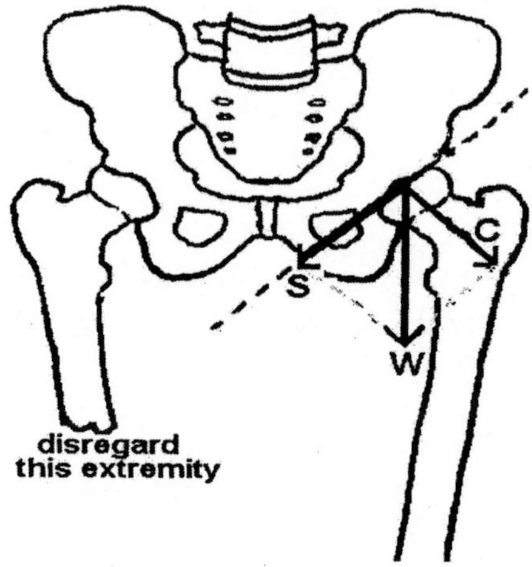

Vector W represents the force of gravity acting on the body mass that is superincumbent to the hip joint. To analyze vector W's effect at the joint surface, we have translated it through space until its point of application lies on the reference line. The vector's exact placement on the reference line is unimportant as long as we neither "tip" (angulate) the vector nor change its magnitude (length) during the translation. Of course, once we move the vector from its original location, we can no longer use it to measure moment arms, but that is not our purpose.

Instead, our purpose is to understand how gravity's force affects the joint surface. To accomplish this, we resolve gravity's force into two component forces, both of which act at right angles to one another:

1. A component that lies at a right angle to the reference line. This is vector C, so named here because it demonstrates how much of gravity's force, acting on the pelvis and superincumbent mass, produces compression between the pelvis and the femoral head.
2. A component that lies directly on the reference line. This is vector S, so named here because it represents a shear force, a force that produces a sliding along the joint surface. This vector's medial direction demonstrates that gravity causes the acetabulum to slide medially on the femoral head.

It takes some practice to learn how long to draw the component vectors. The finished product should look like the figure, with the component vectors drawn just long enough so the original vector is actually their resultant. (Vector resolution is a reciprocal operation to vector composition, much like division is a reciprocal arithmetic operation to multiplication.)

The same analysis clarifies the effects on the hip joint surface of the abductor muscles.

A muscular force's effect on the hip joint surface during unilateral stance

Using the technique of vector resolution, we can analyze the effects that force in the hip abductors (vector A) has on the hip's articular surfaces.

We begin by drawing a red, dashed reference line that approximates the hip joint surface's orientation. The joint surface is curved, so we estimate the orientation of a line that is a tangent to that curved surface.

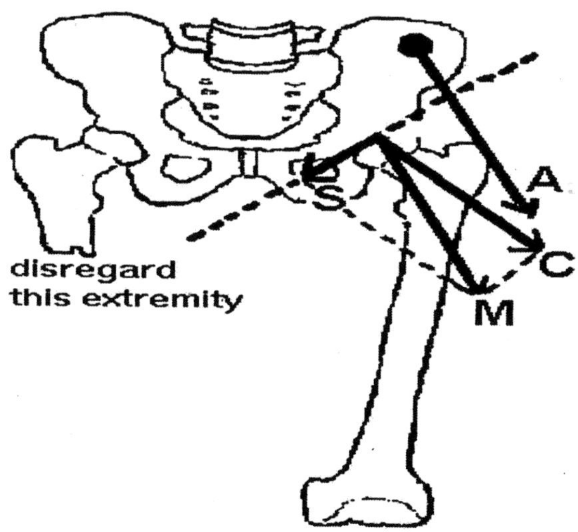

The hip abductors (vector A) act during unilateral stance to oppose the hip adductor moment that gravity produces, and to keep the pelvis level.

We translate vector A through space, neither tipping it nor changing its magnitude, until its point of application rests on the reference line. In its new location (vector M), we resolve it into two component vectors.

One component of the muscle's force (Vector C) compresses the acetabulum into the femur, while the other shear component (Vector S) causes the acetabulum to slide along the surface of the femoral head.

This analysis, along with that of gravity's effect on the hip joint, illustrates how both gravity (body weight) and the hip abductor muscles produce forces that compress the hip joint surface.

Because the abductor muscles' force exceeds that of the superincumbent body weight, most of the compression that the hip joint surface experiences during single limb stance, walking, or running actually comes from muscle action. This explains the curious finding that compressive forces at the hip can equal 2.4 to 2.6 times body weight in unilateral stance, and 4 to 7 times body weight during gait.

The analysis also explains certain behaviors among people whose hip joints are deteriorating due to a degenerative disease like osteoarthritis. An arthritic hip joint's response to joint compression includes inflammation and pain. Individuals seek to decrease hip pain by decreasing joint surface compression.

Because they cannot easily accomplish this by reducing the superincumbent body weight, they reduce instead the abductor muscle activity that produces a large part of the joint compression. They accomplish this in a manner similar to the one people use whey they cannot develop abductor muscle force, by altering their posture and alignment to reduce the moment arm of gravity's force on the hip joint.

This reduces force demands on the hip abductors, thereby reducing the net compressive force on the hip joint surface.

Not only do they adapt by using a lateral trunk lean when they walk, but they benefit from using an assistive device, like a cane, on the side opposite to the painful hip joint.

Newtons Laws of Motion

Adding and resolving forces

In practical biomechanical problems, the limbs or orthoses which are analysed will usually be subjected to a number of forces acting in various directions. Often, we will wish to 'add' these forces together to determine their overall or resultant effect. However, as forces are vectors, that is, they have direction as well as magnitude; they cannot simply be added numerically. If all the forces involved act along the same line they can be added algebraically - that is forces acting in one direction are regarded as positive, whilst those acting in the opposite direction are regarded as negative.

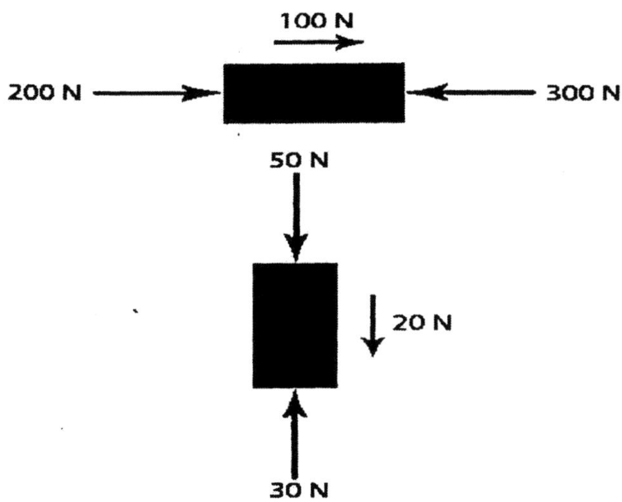

Forces

Forces make things move, stop things moving, or make things change shape. They can either push or pull. In the SI system of units, forces are measured in Newton (N). All forces thus have two characteristics, magnitude and direction, and both need to be stated in order to describe the force fully. Force is a vector quantity, which simply means it has both direction and magnitude.

In Statics we apply the fundamental concepts of mechanics, force and moment, to the analysis of objects which are at rest. A good place to start is with the laws formulated by Newton.

Newton's laws

Sir Isaac Newton in 1687 published three simple laws which together enshrine the fundamental principles of mechanics.

Newton's first law

If an object is at rest it will stay at rest; and if it is moving with a constant speed in a straight line it will continue to do so; as long as no external force acts on it. i.e. If an object is not experiencing the action of an external force it will either keep moving or not move at all.

This law expresses the concept of inertia. The inertia of a body can be described as being its reluctance to start moving, or stop moving once it has started.

At Rest

Constant Velocity

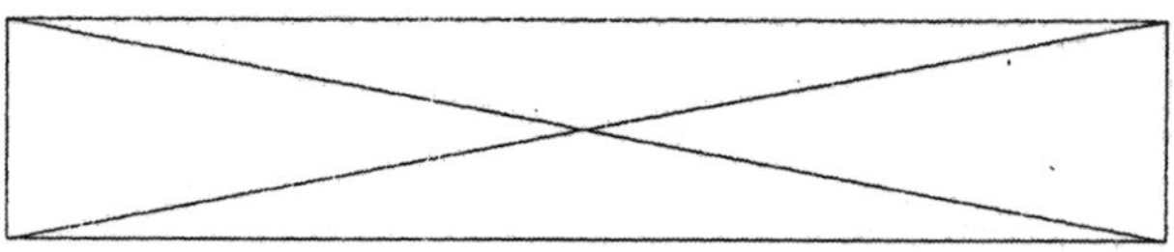

Why does a car slow down when rolling on a flat road?

There are a number of external forces that need to be considered, wind resistance, friction in the bearings of the wheels and axle.

This means we have to be careful to consider all the forces that are acting on an object in order to find out how it is going to move.

Newton's second law

The rate of change of velocity is directly proportional to the applied, external, force acting on the body and takes place in the direction of the force. Therefore forces can either cause an acceleration or deceleration of an object. **Acceleration** is usually define as being positive and **Deceleration** as being negative.

F = ma

F = applied force (N)
m = mass of the body (kg)
a = acceleration of the body (m/s^2)

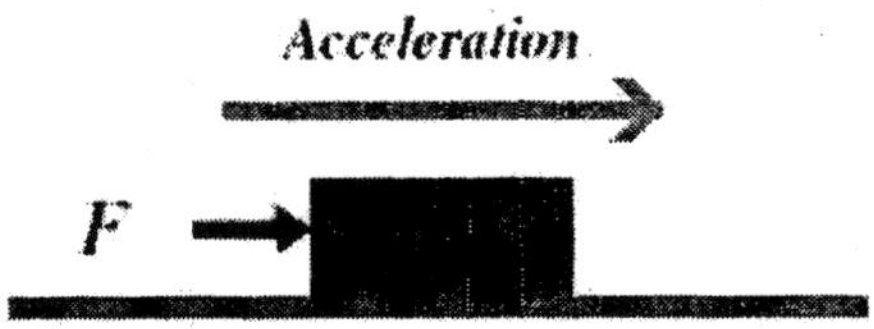

Therefore 1 N is that force which produces an acceleration of 1 m/s2 when it acts on a mass of 1 kg.

Newton' third law

If a body A exerts a force on a body B, then B exerts an equal and opposite directed force on A. This does not mean the forces cancel each other out because they act on two different bodies. The animations below show the action forces and reaction forces.

The runner exerts a force on the ground and receives a reaction force which drives him up and forward. This is known as a **Ground Reaction Force** or **GRF.**

Or

In the case below, a ground reaction force acts from the ground on the ball as the ball bounces.

Mass and Weight

Mass

Mass is the amount of matter an object contains.

This will not change unless the physical properties of the object are changed, wherever the object is moved.

Weight

Weight is a force. This depends on both the mass of the object and the acceleration acting on it. Weight is often interpreted as being the force acting beneath our feet (i.e. scales measure this force, although the never use the correct units which are Newtons).

Therefore a good way to lose weight is to stand in a lift and press the down button. You will lose weight (the ground reaction force will reduce) as the lift accelerates downwards. Unfortunately when the lift comes to a stop you will gain weight again as the lift decelerates downwards.

Another example of the difference between mass and weight is to consider astronauts. When they are in space they are weightless, this does not mean they have gone on an amazing diet, but it does mean that there is no acceleration acting on them.

Weight = mass x acceleration

Acceleration due to Gravity

Wherever you are on planet earth there is acceleration due to gravity acting on you. This does vary a small amount however the value is generally close to 9.81 m/s^2. For the purposes of rough calculations this is often rounded up to 10 m/s^2. It is acceptable to use 10 m/s^2 for the biomechanics covered in this book. However to get the best possible accuracy 9.81 m/s^2 should be used.

Weight = mass x gravity

Or

Weight = m g

Static Equilibrium

The concept of static equilibrium is of great importance in biomechanics as it allows us to calculate forces that are unknown.

Newton's first law tells us that there is no resultant force acting if the body is at rest. i.e. The forces balance.

Therefore if an object is at rest, the sum of the forces on the object, in any direction, must be zero. So when we resolve in a horizontal and vertical direction the resultant force must be zero.

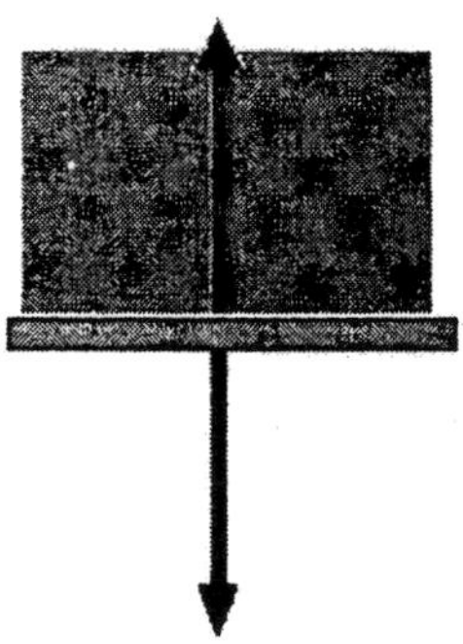

Free Body Analysis

Free body analysis is a technique of looking at and simplifying a problem. The example below shows someone pulling a box along the ground with a piece of string at an angle to the horizontal.

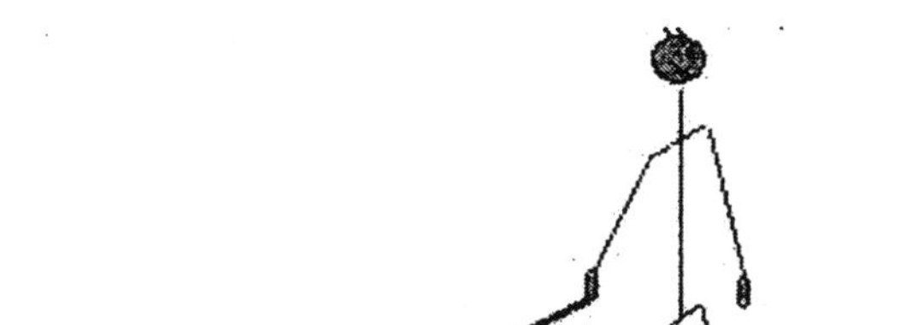

If we now breakdown what force must be acting on the box and form a simplified picture of just the box.

The forces which will be acting are:-

- Tension in the string
- Frictional force
- Weight of the box
- Ground reaction force

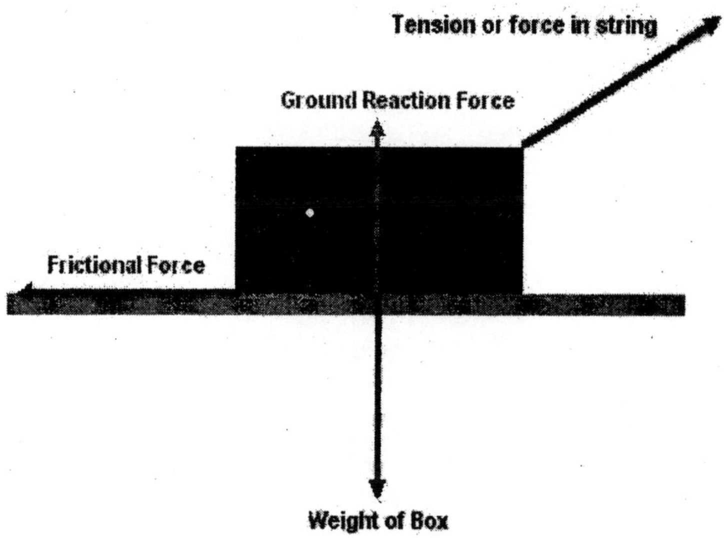

Worked Example: Newton's Laws

Horizontal Forces

Horizontal force in string = 10 cos 30 = 8.66

Therefore 8.66 - 2.66 = mass x acceleration

6 = 4 x a
1.5 m/s2 = a

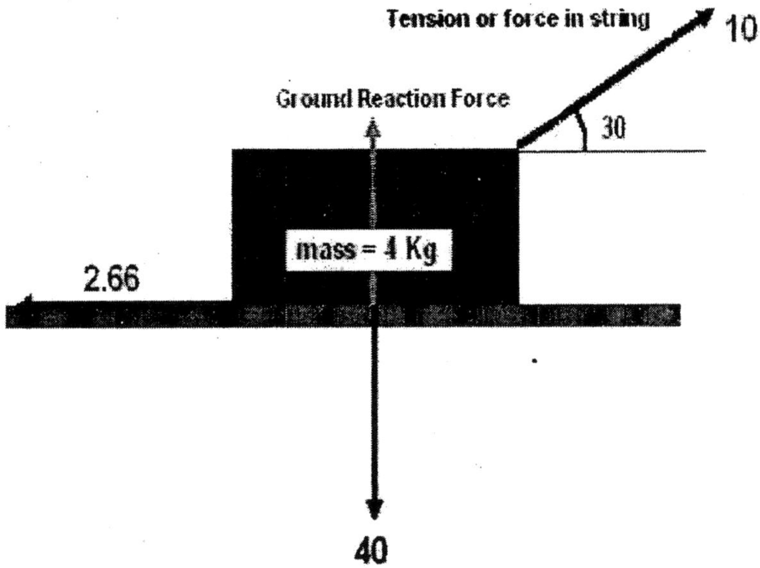

Vertical Forces

Vertical force in string = 10 sin 30 = 5

Ground Reaction Force + 5 - 40 = 0

Ground Reaction Force = 40 - 5 = 35 N

Pressure

Quantitative Assessment of Foot Pressure

What is Pressure?

The unit for pressure is the Pascal (Pa), which is the pressure of one Newton per square meter. Pressure is dependent of the force applied and the area which the force acts through.

Pressure = Force / Area

The Pressure when Standing on two block of different sizes

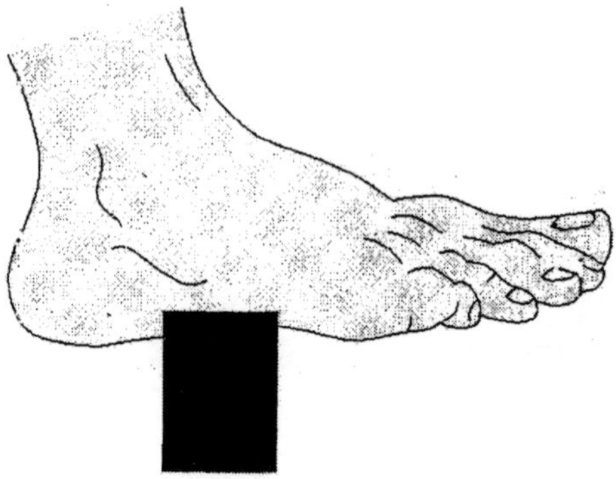

A subject of weight 700 N stands on a 4 cm^2 block

The Area beneath the foot in contact with the block

Area = 0.04 x 0.04 =0.0016 m^2

The Force beneath the foot will be equal to the weight from Newton's third law

Force = 700 N

The Average Pressure between the foot and the block

Pressure = Force / Area

Pressure = 700 / 0.0016 = 437,500 N/m^2 = 437.5 KN/m^2 or Pa

If the subject of weight 700 N now stands on a 2 cm^2 block

The Area beneath the foot in contact with the block

Area = 0.02 x 0.02 =0.0004 m^2

The Force beneath the foot will be equal to the weight from Newton's third law

Force = 700 N

The Average Pressure between the foot and the block

Pressure = Force / Area

Pressure = 700 / 0.0004 = 1750,000 N/m^2 = 1750 KN/m^2 or Pa

E.g., If an individual stands with flat feet they will have lower pressures on the foot than an individual with arched feet as the area over which the force is distributed is larger.

This only considers the average pressure over the whole foot. However load will not be evenly distributed over the whole of the base of the foot, but will be concentrated a various points on the foot.

Friction

What causes Friction?

When the two surfaces meet what happens?

The surfaces in contact weld together microscopically. Then when the objects continue to move against each other the peaks break off.

This leaves fragments which resist the movement and wear down the surfaces.

So where there is friction there is wear. Look at the soles of your shoes.

Static Friction

When a body moves or tries to move over a surface it experiences a frictional force. The frictional surfaces act along a common surface, and are in a direction to oppose the movement.

If at first the pulling force is small, the block does not move.

As the pulling force increases it reaches a point where the block starts to slide.

This indicates that for small values of pulling force the frictional force is equal and opposite, but there is a maximal frictional force that can be brought into play. This is known as the limiting frictional force. When the pulling force is greater than the limiting frictional force the object will accelerate in accordance to Newton's 2nd law.

Laws of Friction

- The frictional force between two surfaces opposes their relative motion.
- Frictional forces are independent of area of contact of the surfaces.
- For two surfaces which have no relative motion the limiting friction is directly proportional to the normal reaction.
- For two surfaces which have relative motion the sliding force is directly proportional to the normal reaction and is approximately independent to the relative velocity of the surfaces.

Frictional force depends on:-

- The normal reaction, how hard the block is pressing down onto the surface, but perpendicular to the surface.
- The roughness of the contact between the two surfaces.

Coefficient of Friction

The frictional force can be shown to be proportional to the normal reaction force by placing increasing loads on a platform and then applying a horizontal force. The force require to move the platform will increase with the loading on the platform. Therefore we can say as the reaction force increases so does the limiting frictional force.

$$F \propto R$$

Where:

F = limiting frictional force
R = normal reaction

Therefore as the normal reaction (R) increases the limiting frictional force (F) would also increase.

The limiting frictional force will vary depending on the materials the two surfaces are made of. Each combination of materials will have its own coefficient of friction given the symbol:

$$\mu$$

So the friction force F, depends on the normal reaction force and the roughness (coefficient of friction) between the two surfaces.

$$F \alpha \mu R$$

Where

F = limiting frictional force
R = normal reaction
μ = coefficient of friction

The animation below shows the frictional force increasing in proportion to the applied force. The object is then pulled along a flat surface at a constant velocity.

The frictional force equals the pulling force as the object is neither accelerating nor decelerating.

Maximum Frictional Force Available

This may be found using the equation below:

Maximum Frictional Force Available = Normal Reaction x Coefficient of Friction

Moments or Torque

When a force acts on a body away from its pivoting point a turning effect is set up. Consider opening and closing a door. You are in fact creating sufficient force to turn the door on its hinges, the force required to do this multiplied by the distance away from the hinges you are pushing is the moment.

A Turning Moment is defined as:-

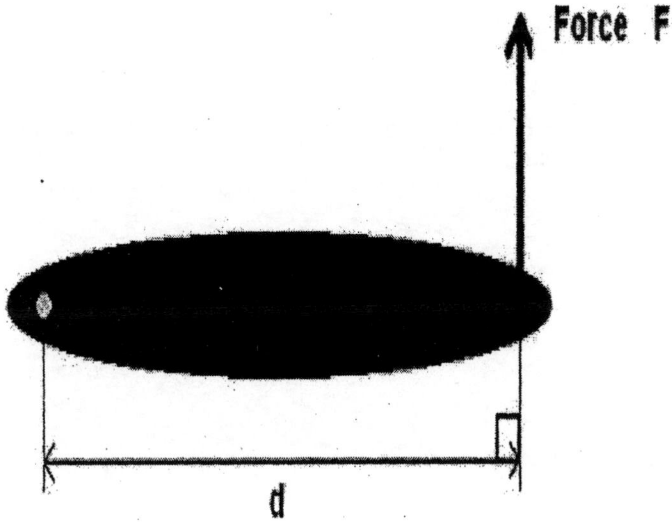

M = F x d

M = Turning Moment
F = The magnitude of force (how hard you push)
d = the perpendicular distance of the line of action of the force away from the centre of rotation.

Balancing Moments

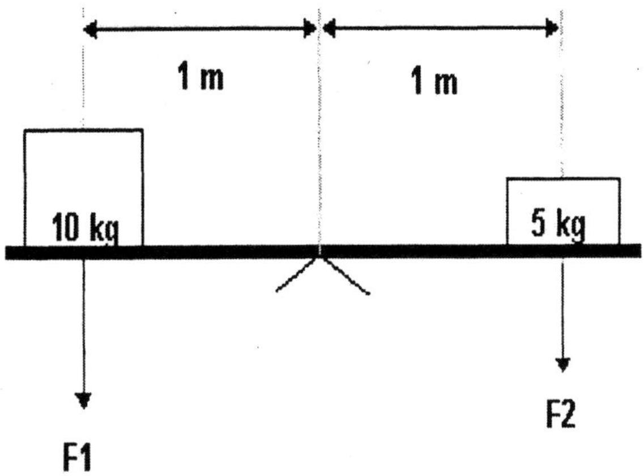

It is clear that the seesaw above does not balance, however if the 10 kg mass was moved so it was half the distance away from the pivot (point of rotation) it would balance.

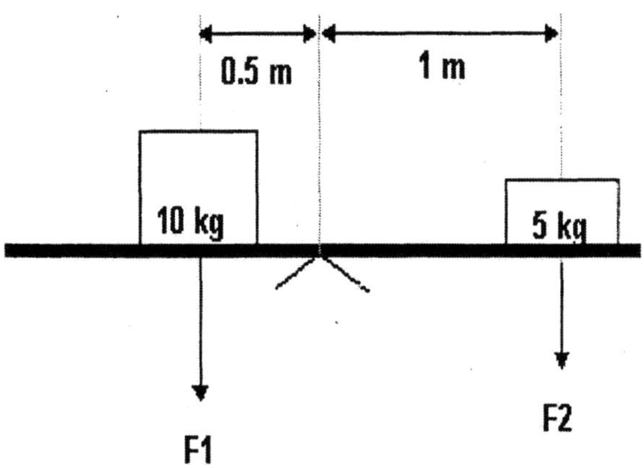

The mathematics

To solve problems with moments we have to consider what the action of each force would be in turn. To do this we consider if it will rotate the object (in this case a seesaw) in a clockwise or anti-clockwise direction. If it is in a clockwise direction it is considered to be in a positive direction, and if anti-clockwise it is considered to be in a negative direction.

Force = mass x acceleration due to gravity

F1 = 10 x 9.81
F1= 98.1 N
(this will try and turn the seesaw anticlockwise)

F2 = 5 x 9.81
F2 = 49.05 N
(this will try and turn the seesaw clockwise)

If the seesaw balances then the sum of the clockwise turning effects and anticlockwise turning effects must be zero. If we say that anticlockwise moments are negative and clockwise are positive then:

Sum of the Moments = - (F1 x 0.5) + (F2 x 1)

Sum of the Moments = - (98.1 x 0.5) + (49.05 x 1) = 0

I.e., the moments cancel out and there is no movement of the see saw.

Vertically

Although there seems to be little effect when we consider the seesaw vertically we have two masses either side giving a total load of 147.15 N downward. From Newton's third law there must be an equal and opposite reaction at the pivot of 147.15 N acting up onto the seesaw.

The Three Lever Arrangements

With Reference to the human body considers that:-

- The force is a muscle force
- The pivot is a joint
- The load is either the weight of the limb or an externally applied force.

First Class Lever

A first class lever is where the pivot is between the load and the force.

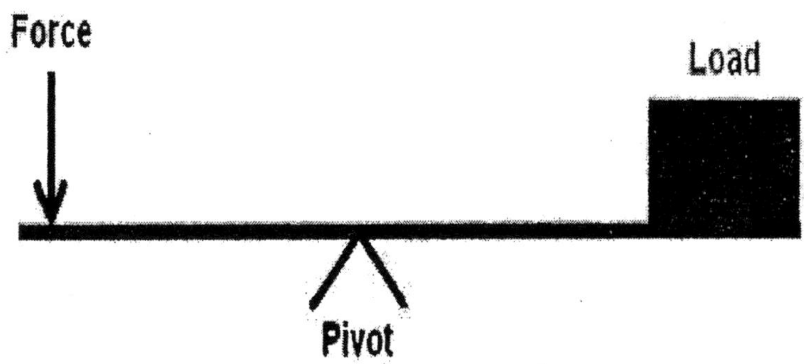

Second Class Lever

A second class lever is where the force is between the load and the pivot.

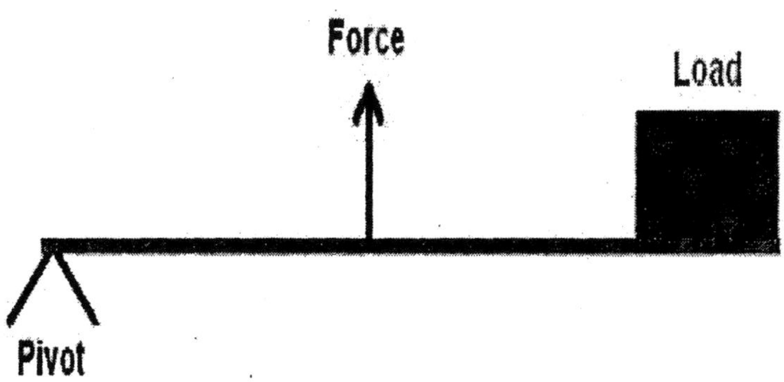

Third Class Lever

A third class lever is where the load is between the force and the pivot.

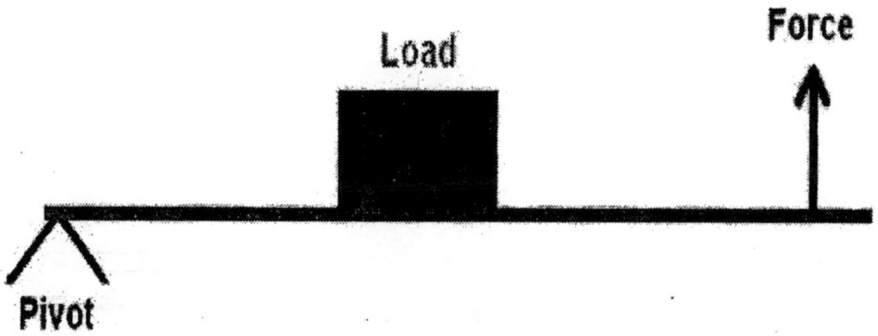

Chapter 2

Forces

Properties of Force

A Force is;

- Push or pull
- Friction
- Blow or impact
- Gravity
- Something that causes or tends to cause a change in the motion or shape of an object or body.

Internal Forces: Forcing originating inside the system.

External Forces: Forces originating outside the system.

Whenever any body or object moves, it does so because some external force has been applied to it.

The Four Properties of a Force

- **Magnitude**: How much force is applied
- **Direction**: The way the force is applied
- **Point of application**: Where the force is applied on the body or system receiving it
- **Line of Action**: The straight line extending through the point of application and extending indefinitely along the direction of the force

Mass: Matter, the stuff of which something is made.

Inertia: A body's resistance to change. The inertia of a body is related to the quantity of mass. The more mass, the more inertia.

The inertia of the leg is greater than the inertia of the arm because the leg has more mass.
Mass/Inertia should not however be synonymous with size.

Weight: The measure of the force with which the earth pulls on the body's mass. A body's mass and weight are directly proportional. The more mass a body has the greater the earth's force of attraction on it, therefore the more the body weighs.

Center of Gravity: The total effect of the force of gravity on a whole body, or system, is as if the force of gravity were concentrated at a single point (CG). In anatomical position, a person's center of gravity is the intersection of the four planes of the body. Balanced point of a system.

Types of Forces

A force is a push or pull acting upon an object as a result of its interaction with another object. There are a variety of types of forces.

Contact Forces	**Action-at-a-Distance Forces**
Frictional Force	Gravitational Force
Tensional Force	Electrical Force
Normal Force	Magnetic Force
Air Resistance Force	
Applied Force	
Spring Force	

These types of individual forces will now be discussed in more detail. To read about each force listed above, continue scrolling through this page. Or to read about an individual force, click on its name from the list below.

- Applied Force
- Gravitational Force
- Normal Force
- Frictional Force
- Air Resistance Force
- Tensional Force
- Spring Force

Type of Force (& Symbol)	Description of Force
Applied Force Fapp	An applied force is a force which is applied to an object by a person or another object. If a person is pushing a desk across the room, then there is an applied force acting upon the object. The applied force is the force exerted on the desk by the person.
Gravity Force (also known as Weight) Fgrav	The force of gravity is the force at which the earth, moon, or other massively large object attracts another object towards itself. By definition, this is the weight of the object. All objects upon earth experience a force of gravity which is directed "downward" towards the center of the earth. The force of gravity on earth is always equal to the weight of the object as found by the equation: **Fgrav = m * g** where g = 9.8 m/s^2 (on Earth) and m = mass (in kg)
Normal Force Fnorm	The normal force is the support force exerted upon an object which is in contact with another stable object. For example, if a book is resting upon a surface, then the surface is exerting an upward force upon the book in order to support the weight of the book. On occasions, a normal force is exerted horizontally between two objects which are in contact with each other.
Friction Force Ffrict	The friction force is the force exerted by a surface as an object moves across it or makes an effort to move across it. The friction force opposes the motion of the object. For example, if a book moves across the surface of a desk, then the desk exerts a friction force in the opposite direction of its motion. Friction results from the two surfaces being pressed together closely, causing intermolecular attractive forces between molecules of different surfaces. As such, friction depends upon the nature of the two surfaces and upon the degree to which they are pressed together. The friction force can be calculated using the equation:

	$F_{frict} = \mu \times F_{norm}$ where μ = coefficient of friction
Air Resistance Force Fair	The air resistance is a special type of frictional force which acts upon objects as they travel through the air. Like all frictional forces, the force of air resistance always opposes the motion of the object. This force will frequently be neglected due to its negligible magnitude. It is most noticeable for objects which travel at high speeds (e.g., a skydiver or a downhill skier) or for objects with large surface areas.
Tensional Force Ftens	The tension is the force which is transmitted through a string, rope, or wire when it is pulled tight by forces acting from each end. The tensional force is directed along the wire and pulls equally on the objects on either end of the wire.
Spring Force Fspring	The spring force is the force exerted by a compressed or stretched spring upon any object which is attached to it. An object which compresses or stretches a spring is always acted upon by a force which restores the object to its rest or equilibrium position. For most springs (specifically, for those which are said to obey "Hooke's Law"), the magnitude of the force is directly proportional to the amount of stretch or compression.

A few further comments should be added about the single force which is a source of much confusion to many students of physics - the force of gravity. The force of gravity acting upon an object is sometimes referred to as the **weight** of an object. Many students of physics confuse weight with mass. The **mass** of an object refers to the amount of matter that is contained by the object; the weight of an object is the force of gravity acting upon that object. Mass is related to "how much *stuff* is there" and weight is related to the pull of the Earth (or any other planet) upon that *stuff*. The mass of an object (measured in kg) will be the same no matter where in the universe those objects are located. Mass is never altered by location, the pull of gravity, speed or even the existence of other forces. For example, a 2-kg object will have a mass of 2 kg whether it is located on Earth, the moon, or Jupiter; its mass will be 2 kg whether it is moving or not (at least for purposes of our study); and its mass will be 2 kg whether it is being pushed or not.

On the other hand, the weight of an object (measured in Newtons) will vary according to where in the universe the object is. Weight depends upon which planet is exerting the force and the distance the object is from the planet. Weight, being equivalent to the force of gravity, is dependent upon the value of **g**. On earth's surface **g** is 9.8 m/s^2 (often approximated as 10 m/s^2). On the moon's surface, **g** is 1.7 m/s^2. Go to another planet, and there will be another **g** value. Furthermore, the g value is inversely proportional to the distance from the center of the planet. So if we were to measure **g** at a distance of 400 km above the earth's surface, then we would find the **g** value to be less than 9.8 m/s^2. Always be cautious of the distinction between mass and weight. It is the source of much confusion for many students of physics.

The meaning of each of these forces will have to be thoroughly understood to successfully proceed through this unit. Ultimately, you must be capable of reading a verbal description of a physical situation and know enough about these forces to recognize their presence (or absence) and to construct a free-body diagram which illustrates their relative magnitude and direction.

Each force act in different way on structures such as bridges, chairs, buildings, in fact any structure. The main examples of forces are shown below. Study the diagram and text and then draw a diagram/pictogram to represent each of these forces.

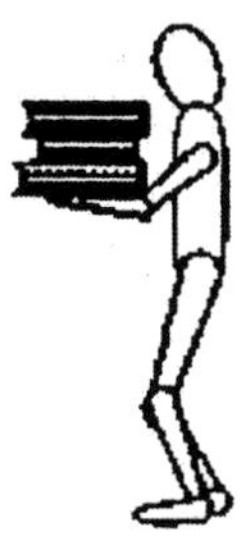

STATIC LOAD (standing still) A good example of this is a person seen on the left. He is holding a stack of books on his back but he is not moving. The force downwards is STATIC.

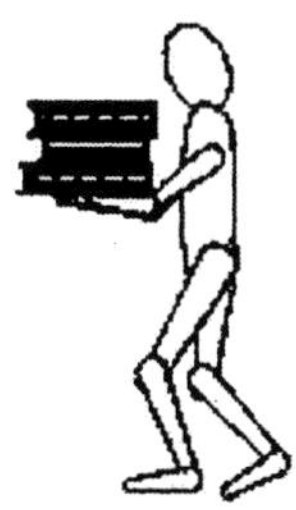

DYNAMIC LOAD (moving) A good example of a dynamic load is the person on the right. He is carrying a weight of books but walking. The force is moving or DYNAMIC.

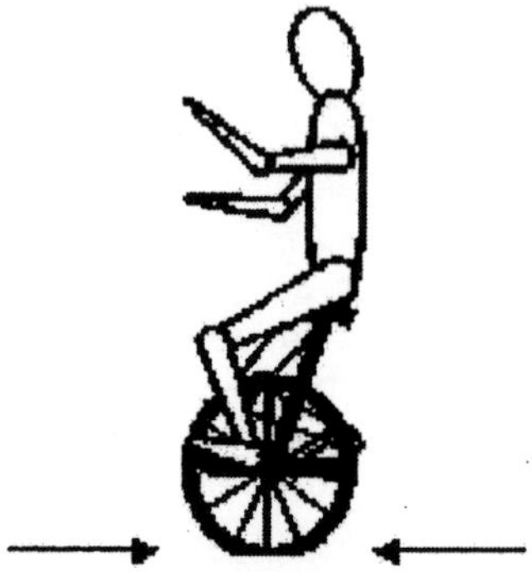

INTERNAL RESISTANCE- The person in the diagram is sat on the mono-bicycle and the air filled tyre is under great pressure. The air pressure inside it pushes back against his/her weight.

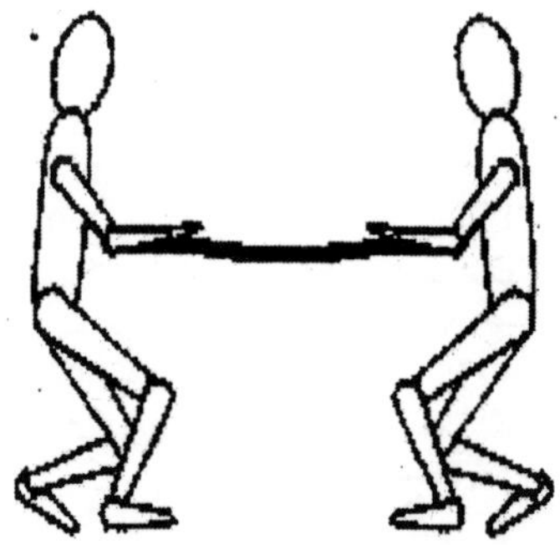

TENSION: The rope is in "tension" as the two people pull on it. This stretching puts the rope in tension.

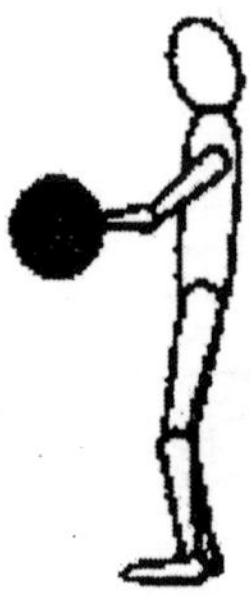

Compression: The weight lifter finds that his body is compressed by the weights he is holding above his head.

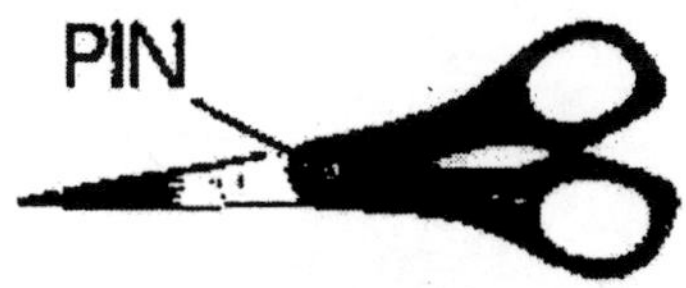

Shear Force: A good example of shear force is seen with a simple scissors. The two handles put force in different directions on the pin that holds the two parts together. The force applied to the pin is called shear force.

Torsion: The plastic ruler is twisted between both hands. The ruler is said to be in a state of torsion.

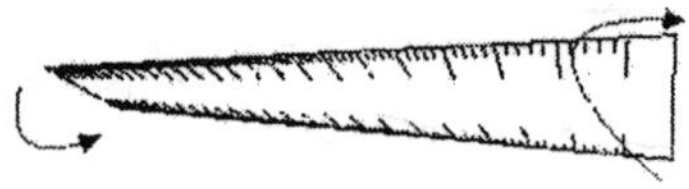

Centripetal Acceleration:

- In order for an object to execute circular motion - even at a constant speed - the object must be accelerating towards the center of rotation. This acceleration is called the centripetal or radial acceleration and has a magnitude of

$$a_c = \frac{v_T^2}{r} = \omega^2 r$$

a_c	= Centripetal acceleration	SI: m/s^2
v_T	= Tangential velocity or speed	SI: m/s
r	= Radius of object's path	SI: m
ω	= Angular velocity	SI: rad/s

Centripetal Force:

- The radial force needed to create this acceleration is call the centripetal force. It is directed towards the center of rotation and has a magnitude of

$$F_c = m a_c = m \frac{v_T^2}{r} = m \omega^2 r$$

- For any object undergoing uniform circular motion, the net force towards the center of rotation must have a value equal the centripetal force.

Centrifugal Force:

- In a frame of reference rotating with an angular velocity ω (omega), the object will be at rest, yet seem to experience a force acting upon it radially outwards equal to $\mathbf{m}\ \omega^2\mathbf{r}$. This is because a rotating frame is a non-inertial frame of reference, i.e. the frame does not move at a constant speed in a straight line, and consequently Newton's First Law does not apply.

It is sometimes useful to move into a frame that is rotating with the system. In this rotating frame, the centripetal force is replaced with a force of the same magnitude acting outwards, which is called the centrifugal force. ("Centrifugal" means "fleeing from the center.") In solving a problem in the rotating frame, the centrifugal force can be treated as though it were another physical force acting on the object with a magnitude $m\ \omega^2 r$ (the same magnitude as the centripetal force) directed radially outwards. Most physicists would advise against doing this, because the centrifugal force is not a real force. I still find it useful in visualizing a problem.

Resistive and Motive Forces

Resistive Forces

Resistive Forces oppose or resist the movement of a system within a frame of reference and they must be external to the system. Resistive forces of a body segment: (help provide stability)

- Tension of muscles
- Connective Tissue
- Contact forces of two parts
- viscosity

Resistive muscular tensions control the speed of segmental movements that we normally take for granted. They are braking forces.

Motive Forces

Forces that cause a change in the way a body segment moves can originate from within the human body or from outside it as long as the forces are external with respect to the segment/system.

- Muscle contraction
- Recoil of stretched connective tissue
- Gravity (always present)

Simultaneous application of Motive and Resistive Forces

When two or more external forces are applied to a system, the system's direction of motion change will reflect the force that wins over the other. The magnitude of the winning force is the difference between the motive and resistive force magnitudes.

First Class Levers

- The axis is located between the motive force and the resistive force
- i.e. teeter-totter
- An example in the body includes the triceps acting to extend the elbow over head

Second Class Levers

- The rotary component of the resistive force is located between the rotary component of the motive force and the axis
- Provides a force advantage for the motive force – therefore less motive force is required to move a greater resistance
- i.e. pushing a wheelbarrow, cracking a nut with a nutcracker
- an example in the body is a push-up where the feet are fixed and act as the axis of rotation, the weight of the body at the center of gravity is the external resistive force and the reaction force of the ground pushing against the hands is the external motive force

Third Class Levers

- The rotary component of the motive force is located between the axis and the rotary component of the resistive force
- i.e. shoveling, batting in baseball
- This class comprises most of the levers found within the musculoskeletal system because the muscle attachments are closer to the joint axis of rotation than are the resistances they are moving

The gravitational force

The gravitational force is based on and proportional to an object's masses. A larger object of similar density will 'pull' harder on a smaller object of the same density. It was Isaac Newton who described his 'universal law of gravitation' in 1666.

$$F_G = G\,(mM/r^2)$$

Where:

F_G = the gravitational force
G = the gravitational constant ($=6.67\times10^{-11}$ Nm^2/kg^2)
m = mass of object
M = mass of the Earth
r = distance between the center of the two masses m and M.

From all four basic forces gravity is by far the weakest at short distances. At a small scale at the level of subatomic particles, atoms, molecules, and even biological cells both nuclear forces and the electrostatic force are the dominating players. However, at a longer distance both the nuclear forces are reduced to zero, and only the electrostatic and the gravitational forces remain of importance. At even longer distances only the force of gravity prevails.

The dominance of gravity is one of the most obvious phenomena seen in our solar system. It is gravity that keeps the planets orbiting our Sun, gravity keeps the Moon rotating around the Earth, but gravity is also the main enemy of our precious china and glassware!

All the forces we see and experience around us, like our muscle force, the hydraulic force of car brakes, the frictional force when sliding, the elastic force, the force that the Earth atmosphere exerts on a barometer, electrical force that starts a car engine, etc., etc., etc., are forces deriving from these four basic forces as described above.

Work, energy, and power

WORK involves the application of a force over a distance.

Therefore, we measure work in terms of a:

- FORCE (F) acting over a straight line DISTANCE (d).

$$W=Fd$$

- MOMENT of force (M) acting over an arc (of length r) whose center is an axis of rotation

$$W=Mr$$

In either case, work is measured in units like foot*lbs. or N*m.

Because ENERGY (E) is the capacity to do WORK, we measure energy and work in the same units (foot*lbs. or N*m).

E=Fd for "straight-line" work

E=Mr for work around an axis of rotation

POWER (P) is the rate of energy generation (or absorption) *over time*:

$$P = E/t$$

Power's SI unit of measurement is the Watt, representing the generation or absorption of energy at the rate of 1 Joule/sec. Power's unit of measurement in the English system is the horsepower, which is equivalent to 735.7 Watts.

For translational motions:	for rotational motions:
P = Fd/t	**P = Mr/t**

If, in the equation for rotational motion, which includes motion around a joint axis, we substitute:

$$w=r/t$$

for angular velocity (measured in degrees or radians per second), we obtain the familiar equation for JOINT POWER:

$$P=Mw$$

so that JOINT POWER is the product of:

- M (joint moment) and
- w (joint angular velocity.)

Joint Moments

Muscles produce moments of force across joints during the walking cycle. (Other soft tissues, like ligaments, can also produce forces and moments when they are elongated.)

These figures show typical moments at the hip, knee, and ankle during the gait cycle. The support moment is the sum of the extensor moments.

Calculation of joint moments is complex, but is validated by the moments' excellent correspondence with normal muscle activity during gait.

Joint moments are calculated using sophisticated laboratory equipment and computer programs. To understand their derivation, and their importance to clinical gait analysis, consider an observed joint movement represents the effect of the *total moment* that acts at the joint at that instant during the gait cycle.

The total moment at a joint is calculated as the product of two measurable quantities:

1. the joint segments' moments of inertia, which involves knowing thee segments' masses and lengths
2. the joint's angular acceleration

The instantaneous total moment is the *sum* of individual moments produced by:

- ground reaction forces
- joint reaction forces
- muscle and soft tissue forces that produce the joint moment

ground reaction moment
+ joint reaction moment
+ (internal) joint moment
= total moment

We can calculate the ground reaction and joint reaction moments if we also have information on ground reaction forces (from forceplate data) and segmental velocities.

We can then calculate the joint moment as a residual:

total moment
- ground reaction moment
- joint reaction moment
= *joint moment*

We use calculated joint moments to calculate and understand joint power

Energy and power during the gait cycle

Power is Energy / time, the rate at which energy

- Is created (positive power)
- Or absorbed (negative power)

Structures in the body that can generate or absorb energy include

- Muscles
- Other soft tissue

Power is measured in Watts or Joules/second.

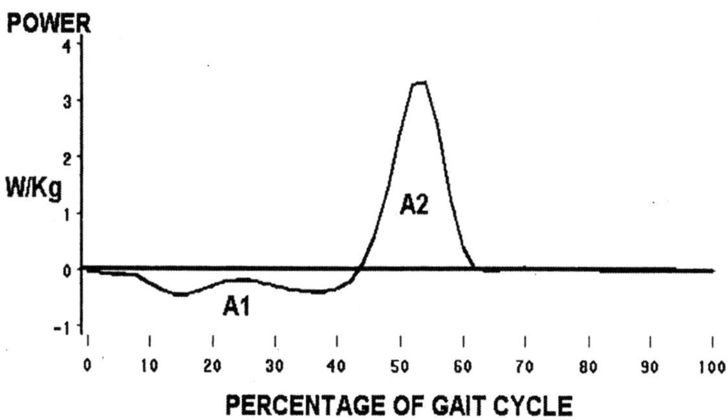

These graphs summarize power at the hip, knee and ankle during normal gait.

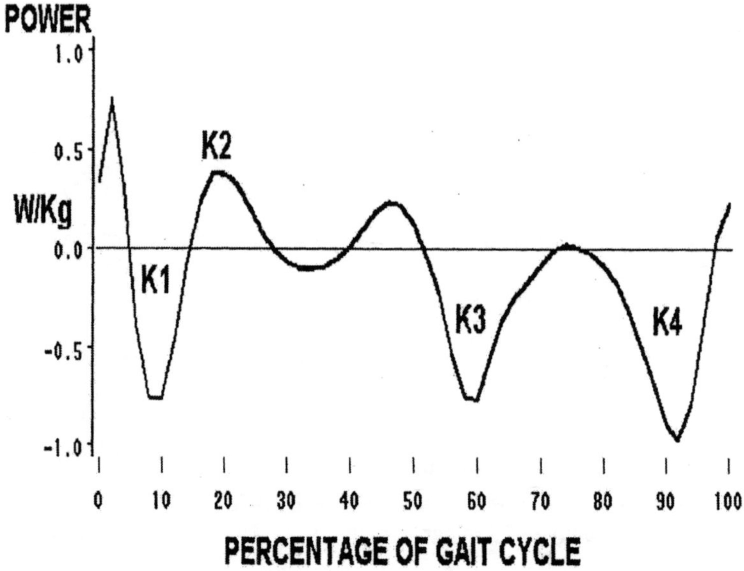

Power is positive when the body generates energy through concentric muscle activity.

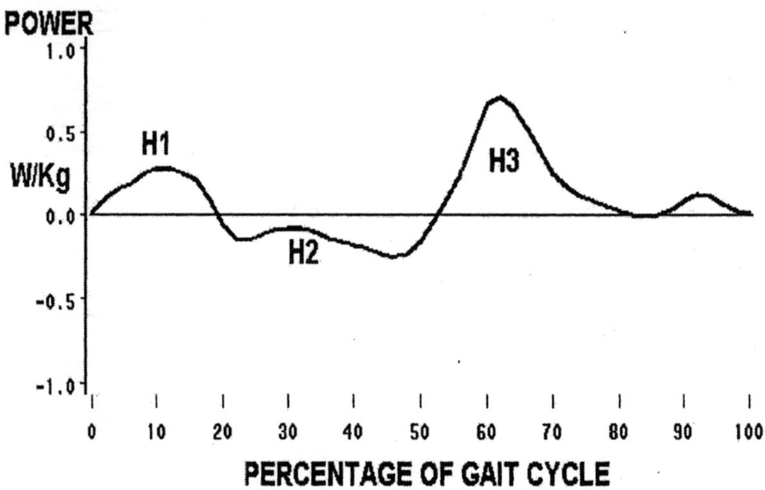

Power is negative when the body absorbs energy through eccentric muscle activity or elongation of soft tissue.

POWER CURVE FOR THE ANKLE JOINT

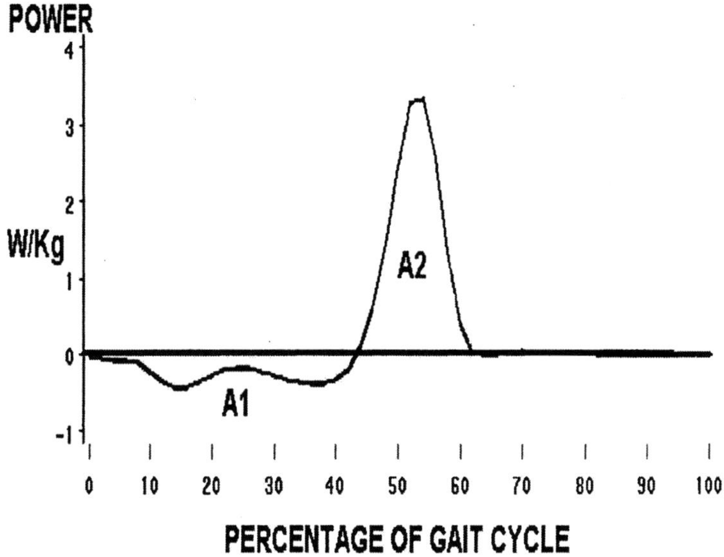

A1: a region of negative power, corresponding to eccentric plantar flexor activity at the ankle during midstance and terminal stance.

A2: a region of positive power, corresponding to the concentric burst of propulsive plantar flexor activity during preswing.

Power Curve for the Knee Joint

K1: a region of negative power, corresponding to eccentric knee extensor activity at during loading response.

K2: a region of positive power, corresponding to concentric knee extensor activity during midstance. This is followed by a period of negligible joint power during that period of time when the ground reaction force stabilizes the knee in extension.

K3: a region of negative power, corresponding to eccentric activity in the rectus femoris during preswing. At normal or slightly faster walking speeds, rectus femoris controls knee flexion.

K4: a region of negative power, corresponding to eccentric activity in the hamstrings during terminal swing.

Power Curve for the Hip Joint

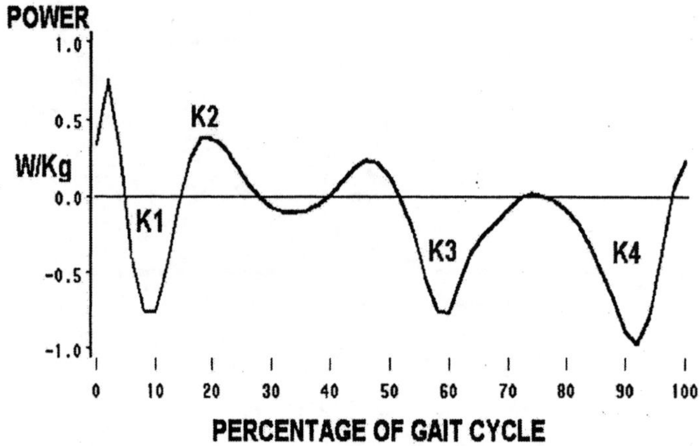

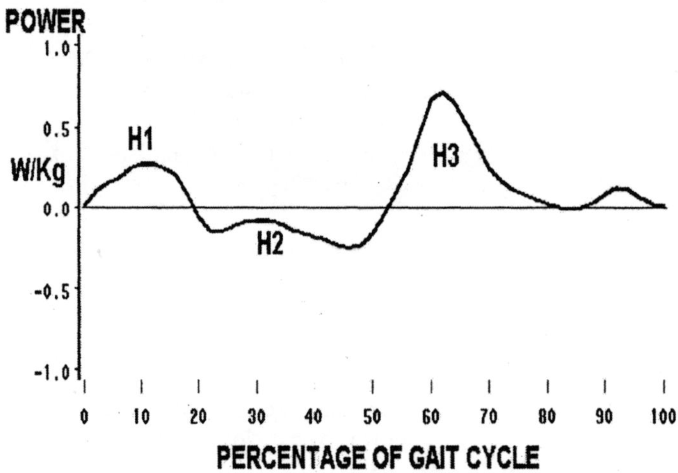

H1: a small region of positive power, not always present, which corresponds to concentric hip extensor activity during loading response.

H2: a region of negative power, corresponding to eccentric hip flexor activity during midstance.

H3: a region of positive power, corresponding to concentric activity in the hip flexors during preswing and intial swing. Sometimes called "pull off," this is the muscular system's second largest contribution of propulsive power during the gait cycle.

Calculation of Joint Power

This figure simultaneously graphs three quantities against percentage of the gait cycle (on the horizontal axis):

1. joint angle

   The first curve's slope at any point in the gait cycle reflects the joint's angular velocity (w).

2. joint moment (M)
3. joint power (P)

At that instant during the gait cycle indicated by the bold vertical line, joint power is the product of joint moment and joint angular velocity.

$$P=M\omega$$

Derivation of formula

Definitions of these and other terms related to kinetics

Power can be a negative or positive quantity

When the muscle moment of force (M) and the direction of joint movement (ω) are the same at a particular joint:

- power is a positive quantity
- energy is generated by concentric action in muscles crossing that joint.

When M and ω are in opposite directions:

- power is a negative quantity
- energy is absorbed in eccentric muscle action and/or elongation of other soft tissue crossing the joint.

Length-Tension Properties Of Muscle

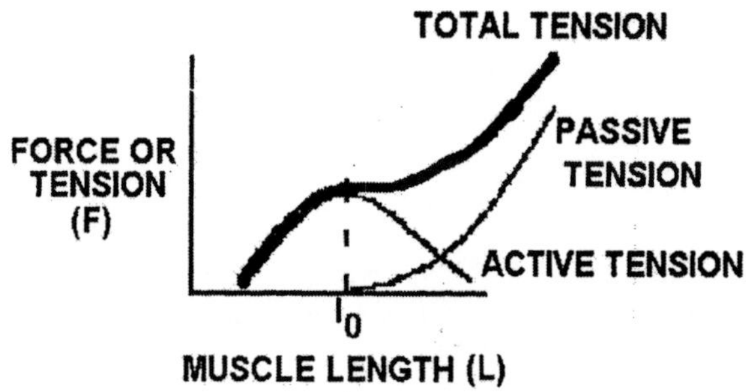

A muscle's length-tension curve illustrates how its force comes from two sources:

- Active tension derives from the interaction between myosin and actin active tension.
- Passive tension can develop in the muscle's complex connective tissue.

Length-tension curves appear in other forms, including force-angle curves and stress-strain curves. All the curves share the same characteristic shape, because the variables graphed on the x and y axes are just scaled versions of length and force.

Stress-strain curves: Stress, a measure of force per area, replaces force on the y-axis. Strain, an expression of the percentage of elongation beyond resting length, replaces absolute length on the x-axis.

Force-angle curves: Joint angle replaces length as the x-axis variable. To use a flexor muscle group as an example, flexors are short when the joint is flexed and elongated when the joint is extended.

Moment-angle curves: As long as a muscle's moment arm is relatively constant throughout the range of motion of the joint that the muscle crosses, then the muscle's moment-angle curve has a shape that is similar to that of its force-angle curve.

Development of passive (viscoelastic) force

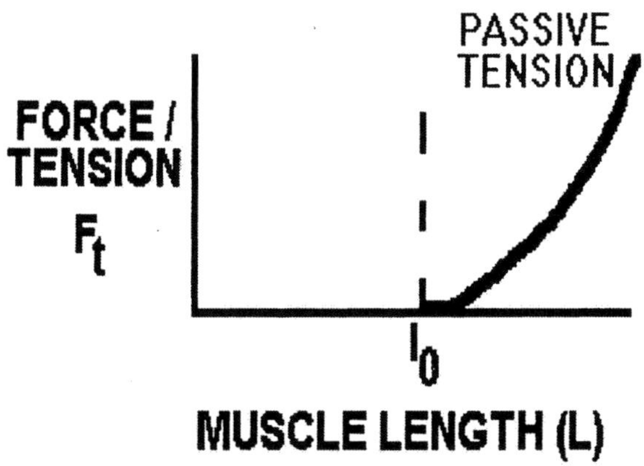

Human tissues, including muscles, behave like springs; they are elastic.

At lengths greater than their resting length (l_0), they develop tension or force. This force is passive, since it exists whether or not the muscle is active.

Passive force, like active force, acts in a direction from the muscle's points of attachment toward its center.

Elasticity or Stiffness

Different muscles demonstrate different passive properties. Some are stiffer than others, that is, they develop more force during a given amount of elongation.

In this figure of muscles' passive stress-strain curves, the stiffer the muscle, the steeper its curves' slope.

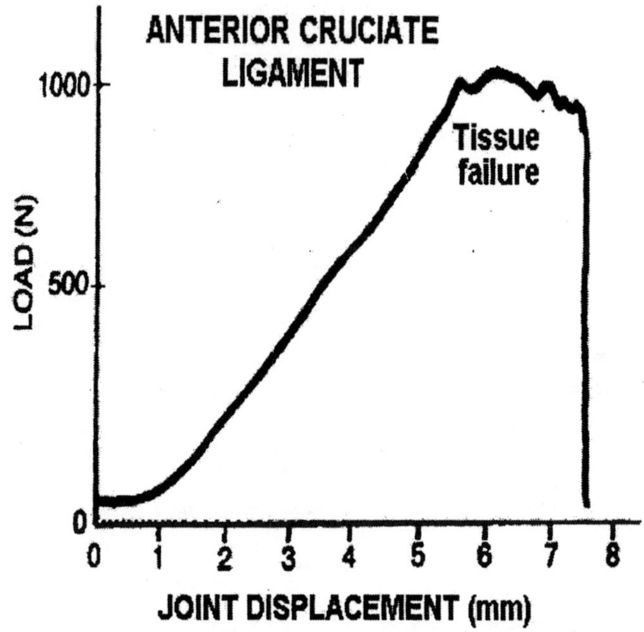

The distinctive stiffness properties of any soft tissue are illustrated by its length-tension curve. The knee's anterior cruciate ligament has a distinct length-tension curve.

Viscosity or Damping Properties

In addition to displaying the property of elasticity, many tissues display viscosity, a resistance to flow. Viscous materials resist elongation more at higher rates of elongation. Highly viscous fluids are "thick" and flow more slowly than "thinner," less viscous fluids.

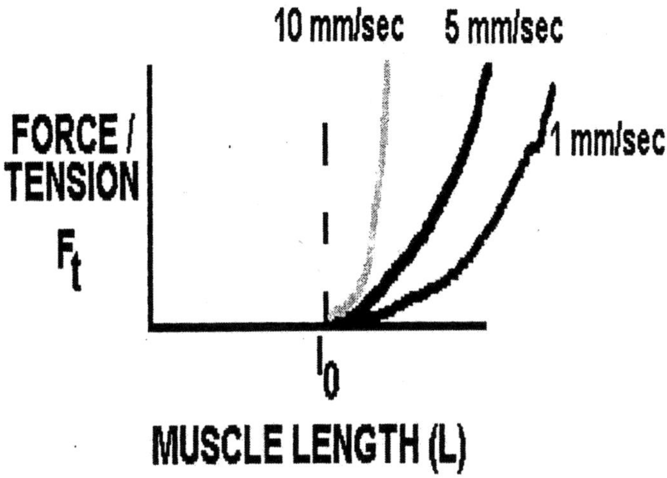

The passive length-tension curve of a viscous material has a slope that changes, increasing as the velocity of elongation increases. The faster the rate of elongation, the stiffer the material's behavior.

Three Sources of Stiffness in Muscle

I. Intrinsic muscle stiffness
   - connective tissue has its own length-tension properties
   - cross-bridges in inactive actin-myosin produce thixotropy, so that a muscle's stiffness depends on its recent movement history.

II. Stiffness due to voluntary muscle activity

III. Reflex stiffness

Development of active force
(or tension):

- Active muscle force is proportional to number of active actin/myosin binding sites.
- The number of sites available for actin/myosin binding depends on the muscle's length.

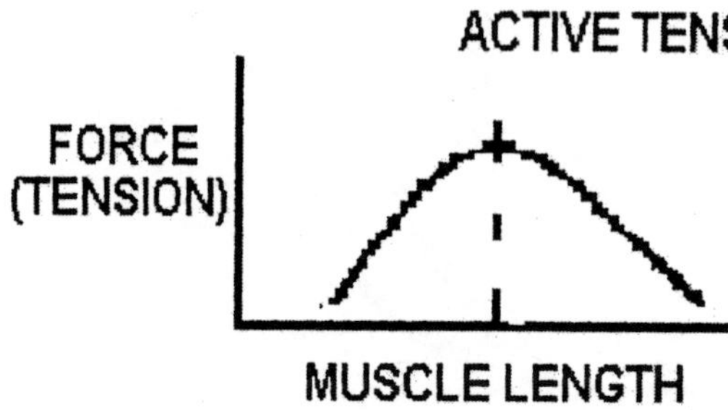

- As the muscle shortens, the increasing overlap of actin and myosin chains leaves relatively few additional binding sites.
- As the muscle is elongated, decreasing overlap of actin and myosin chains provides relatively few binding sites.
- The greatest number of actin-myosin binding sites are available when the muscle fiber is at an intermediate length

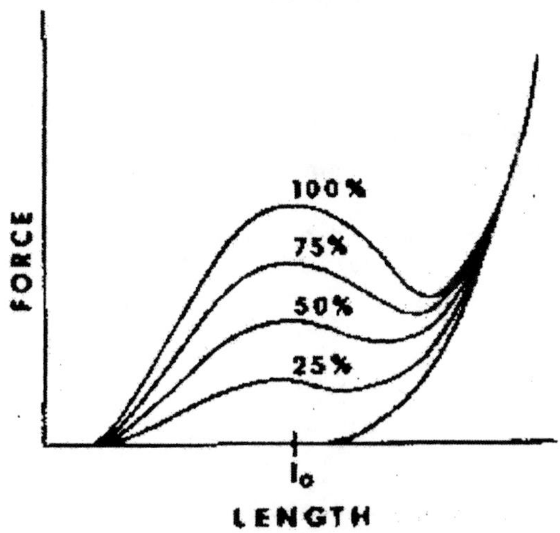

Therefore, the active length-tension curve is dome-shaped. The curve's amplitude (the height of the dome) varies with the amount of active force that the muscle's motor units generate. This graph shows the curve at various percentages of motor unit activation.

The active length-tension curve is theoretical; we can't measure it directly. We obtain the curve by subtracting a passive length-tension curve from a length-tension curve that displays the muscle's isometric force development at different lengths.

Electromyography (EMG)

Purposes:

- Kinesiological EMG
  - functional anatomy
  - force development
  - reflex connections of muscles.
- Diagnostic EMG)
  - strength-duration curves to test nerve and muscle integrity
  - nerve conduction velocity to test for nerve damage / compression
  - firing characteristics of motor neurons and motor units, including analysis of motor unit action potentials (muaps) to detect signs of pathology such as fibrillation potentials and positive sharp waves

The circuit:

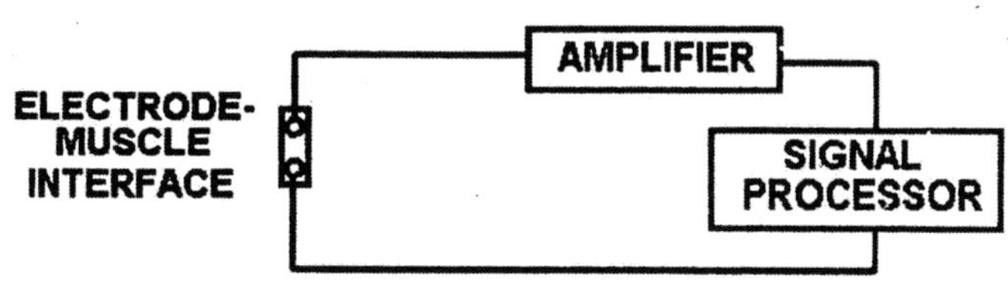

The raw EMG signal:

A voltage difference or difference in electrical potential (E=Ir) measured between recording electrodes

The signal's origins include electrical activity in various tissues:

Potentials in motor units of muscle fibers (muap)

Motor neuron action potential produces an end plate potential

End plate potential directly depolarizes muscle membrane near muscle fiber's center

Depolarization wave travels from muscle's surface along transverse tubules into fiber's interior

Depolarization travels simultaneously along membrane's surface by local current flow, creating a train of bipoles +/-.

The signal is detected by electrodes:

	indwelling • needle • fine wire	surface (Ag-AgCl)
surface area	Large area behaves like a string of point electrodes; each 'point' picks up the same signal, slightly delayed in time; the sum is a longer duration waveform.	small area picks up more discrete signals without producing long duration waveform
pick up zone	limited to 0.5 cm to 1.5 cm; can record only from superficial muscles	necessary for recording from deep muscles
"cross talk" (pickup of signals from adjacent	more common	less common

muscles)		
choice of electrode placement	for electrode to detect a muap, it must travel in a direction such that the distance between impuse and electrode changes Therefore, electrodes should be aligned with expected direction of impulse (or aligned perpendicular to impulses that should be excluded)	

Signal processing and amplification

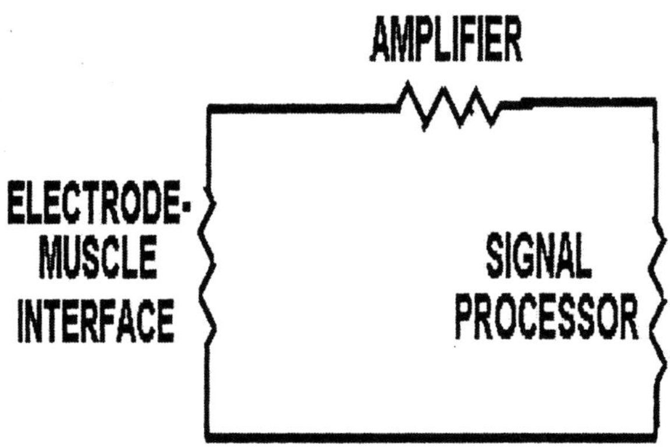

1. Rectification

   Because the raw signal is biphasic, its mean value is zero. The rectifier allows current flow in only one direction, and so "flips" the signal's negative content across the zero axis, making the whole signal positive.

2. Filtering and linear envelope detection

   EMG is actually a composite of many signals, as well as some noise. These voltages also rise and fall at various rates or frequencies, forming a frequency spectrum. Circuits filter the composite signal and eliminate unwanted and meaningless electrical noise like movement artifact. Because most EMG exists in a frequency range between 20 and 200 Hz, and because movement artifacts have frequencies less than 10 Hz, that is the cutoff frequency frequently employed in "high-pass" filters. The

3. Integration

calculating the area under the linear envelope, a quantity analogous to electrical work or energy.

4. Amplification

single muaps have amplitude of 100 microvolts
signals detected by surface electrodes are in range of 5 mV
signals detected by indwelling electrodes are in range of 10 mV

Amplifier impedance

Must be considerably higher than the impedance of the electrode/skin or electrode/muscle interfaces. Since indwelling electrodes have very high impedances (due to low surface area), very high amplifier impedances are necessary.

Common mode rejection

Even when leads are shorted together, a signal of 20 - 50 micro-volts may result from ambient electromagnetic energy, induced by nearby machinery or electrical lines. The body itself is like an antenna that picks up ambient electromagnetic signals, including the 60 Hz signal from ordinary house current. This "hum" is in the middle of EMG frequency range; we can't filter it.

Outcome measures:

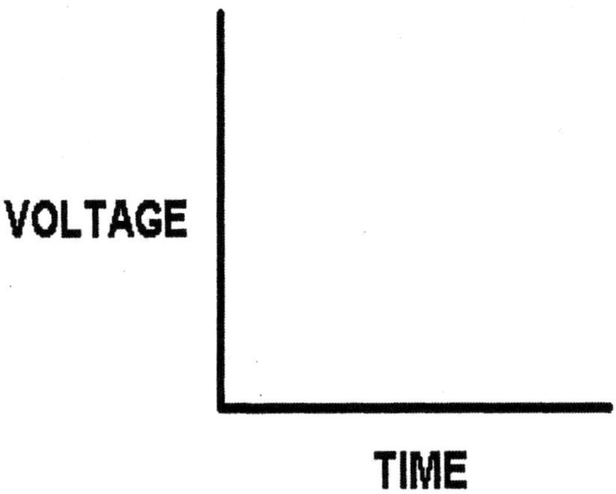

- Vertical axis (voltage)
- Rate of rise of voltage
- Peak amplitude

Horizontal Axis (time)

timing (percent on/off; on/off ratio)
duration (sec; percent of cycle)
coactivation (percent of cycle)
Area under the curve (related to force)

Ellaway's cumulative sum histogram technique:

$$S_i = \sum x_i - \bar{X}$$

Where S_i is the cumulative sum up to sample i, X is the mean voltage over the trial, and x_i is the voltage at sample i.

Frequency analysis or spectral analysis

Kinematic analyses of Gait

Kinematic measures of gait

Kinematic variables describe the extent, speed, and direction of movement of joints or body segments

- Goniometric analysis
- Observational gait analysis
- Stride analysis
    - step length
    - stride length
    - velocity
    - cadence

Summary of gait kinematics

The chart summarizes the kinematic interactions that occur during the gait cycle. The chart's rows distinguish between stance and swing phases. The columns are mapped to information about the relevant joints and segments.

The determinants of normal and pathological gait

Features of the movement pattern that minimizes displacement in the body's center of gravity during gait:

1. Pelvic Rotation
2. Lateral Pelvic Tilt (Drop)
3. Knee Flexion in Stance
4. Knee Ankle Foot Interactions
5. Knee Ankle Foot Interactions
6. Physiological Genu Valgus

	%	EVENTS	LOWER LIMB	KNEE JOINT	ANKLE JOINT	SUBTALAR JOINT	MIDTARSAL JOINT
STANCE		I.C. / foot flat	medial rotation	flexion	plantar flexion	pronation	free motion
	20	midstance	lateral rotation	extension	dorsi-flexion	supination	restricted
	40	heel rise		flexion			
					plantar flexion		
SWING	60	toe-off	medial rotation		dorsi-flexion		
	80			extension			
	100	I.C.					

Examples of how these kinematic features produce an efficient walking pattern:

- During double limb support, that time when the center of gravity is at its lowest point, joint angles in both lower extremities are such that their effective lengths are maximized. Additionally, the pelvis is rotated forward on the side where the limb is in loading response, and backward on the limb which is in preswing. This functional lengthening of the limbs minimizes the vertical drop in the center of gravity.

- During midstance and midswing, when the center of gravity is highest, the stance limb's hip, knee, and ankle are all flexed 5 degrees. In addition, the pelvis is tilted downward laterally toward the swing limb. This minimizes the center of gravity's upward excursion, keeping it lower than if the individual were standing erect.
- The six "determinants" are logically appealing, because they help us focus on a relatively small number of critical factors from among the many degrees of mechanical freedom that are possible during walking. However, very recent research questions whether the determinants are important, at least for the reasons that Inman and Saunders proposed:

CENTER OF GRAVITY DISPLACEMENTS

During ambulation, the body's center of gravity is propelled forward. However it also moves vertically and laterally; we presume a gait pattern to be energy efficient to the extent that it minimizes vertical and lateral displacements.

I. Vertical displacement of COG

Viewed in the sagittal plane, the *vertical displacement* of the center of gravity traces a smooth sinusoidal curve. This curve's amplitude in the normal adult male is approximately 5 cm or 2 inches. The center of gravity moves vertically through two full oscillations during each gait cycle, so that the curve has two peaks and two troughs.

- The low points or troughs in the sinusoidal pathway occur during the gait cycle's two periods of double limb support (loading response and preswing). The depth of the troughs is limited by:
  - Pelvic rotation
  - Knee-ankle-foot interactions
- The high points or peaks occur at midstance and again at midswing. The height of these peaks is limited by:
  - Lateral pelvic tilt (drop)
  - Knee flexion in stance

II. Lateral displacement of COG

The center of gravity also oscillates *laterally* during ambulation. The total lateral displacement traces a sinusoidal curve with an amplitude of approximately 6 centimeters or 2.5 inches. The greatest lateral excursion of the center of gravity occurs at the end of midstance. Thus, only one full lateral oscillation of the center of gravity (to the right and left) occurs during a gait cycle. The amplitude of this lateral excursion is limited by a structural feature in the lower extremities, namely genu valgus.

Observational gait analysis

Although observational gait analysis is the therapist's primary clinical tool for describing the quality of a patient's walking pattern, it can be extremely unreliable. Attempts to systematize observational gait analysis and to maximize its reliability (Krebs, Edelstein, & Fishman, 1985; Eastlack, Arvidson, & Snyder-Mackler, 1991) have led therapists to certain conclusions:

- Binary scoring:

  Rating of gait deviations as "mild," "moderate," or "severe" is unreliable; therapists display low rates of agreement in making these judgements. Agreement is much higher when therapists use a binary scale, one with only two categories, like "present" or "absent."

- Focus on slow moving segments

  Therapists agree more often regarding body segments which move slowly. Observational analysis is more reliable when it focuses on proximal segments instead of distal segments, and on stance phase events instead of swing phase events.

- Focus on sagittal plane, then on frontal plane

  Therapists are most reliable in judging gait patterns from the side and from behind or in front. They are extremely unreliable in judging movements which involve rotation of the LE joints.

Stride analysis

The stride analysis variables most commonly used to describe a gait pattern:

- *Step length* is the distance between the point of initial contact of one foot and the point of initial contact of the opposite foot. In normal gait, right and left step lengths are similar.
- *Stride length* is the distance between successive points of initial contact of the same foot. Right and left stride lengths are normally equal.
- *Cadence* or walking rate is calculated in steps per minute.
- *Velocity*, the product of cadence and step length, is expressed in units of distance per time. "Free speed" refers to the individual's comfortable walking speed. Since individuals walk at different speeds depending on the situation, normal velocity values are somewhat arbitrary.
- *Walking base* is the sum of the perpendicular distances from the points of initial contact of the right and left feet to the line of forward progression.
- *Foot angle* or toe out describes an angle between the line of progression and a line drawn between the midpoints of the calcaneus and the second metatarsal head.

TABLE - MEAN STRIDE ANALYSIS VARIABLES

	Males	**Females**
Step Length (cm)	79	66
Stride Length (cm)	158	132
Cadence (steps/min)	117 (60-132)	117 (60 132
Velocity (m/sec)	1.54	1.31
Walking Base (cm)	8.1	7.1
Foot angle	7	6

Values for men adapted from Murray, Drought, & Kory (1964).

Stance Phase

- Loading Response

  (0 to 10 percent of the gait cycle, the period from initial contact until contralateral toe off)

- Midstance and Terminal Stance

  (from 10 to 50 percent of the gait cycle, ending when the opposite foot contacts the ground)

- Preswing

  (50 to 60 percent of the gait cycle, ending when the foot leaves the ground)

Swing Phase (60 to 100 percent of the gait cycle)

- Pelvis rotates forward and entire lower limb rotates internally.
- Ankle dorsiflexes ankle and knee is flexed.
- STJ pronation / supination is variable.

LOADING RESPONSE

Internal rotation of LE persists from swing phase

- Tibia rotates further/faster than femur, resulting in relative tibial internal rotation.
- Tibial internal rotation permits knee flexion.
- Tibia-fibula and talus rotate together at mortise-like ankle joint.
- Subtalar joint pronates

Midstance and Terminal Stance

Relative backward pelvic rotation and external rotation of entire lower extremity

(This involves an external rotation of the entire lower limb with respect to the line of progress)

- Tibia rotates further/faster than femur, resulting in relative external tibial rotation (relative internal femoral rotation), facilitating knee screw-home/extension
- Tibia-fibula and talus rotate together at mortise-like ankle joint.
- Subtalar joint supinates

Chapter 3

Analysis of Motion

Axis Alignment

In motion analysis, it is advantageous to align a global axis (an axis of the global reference frame) with the direction of motion because it will simplify the data analysis substantially. The global reference frame is initially fixed to the calibration frame.

In other words, one can align a horizontal axis of the global reference frame with the direction of motion through careful placement of the calibration frame. If the calibration frame has cubic or hexahedral shape, this should be fairly easy.

In the survey method, on the other hand, one can place two range poles along the X axis and use one as the origin pole and the other as the X-axis pole. The real-life coordinates of the control points based on this reference frame setup can be easily obtained.

Careful placement of the calibration frame is sufficient in most cases but there are some circumstances in which one must take additional measures to accurately define the global reference frame.

One simple but flexible approach is to use the so-called additional points.

The Additional Point Strategies in 3-D Analysis

One can place up to 3 additional markers in the field of view in addition to the control points during the camera calibration to define the orientation of the global reference frame.

There are three possible strategies in the 3-D analysis:

No. of Additional Points	Axis Transformation Strategy
1	Translation only
2	1-Axis Rotation + Translation
3	2-Axis Rotation + Translation

1-Point Method

This method can be used when one needs to move the origin of the reference frame (to translate the reference frame) (Figure 1).

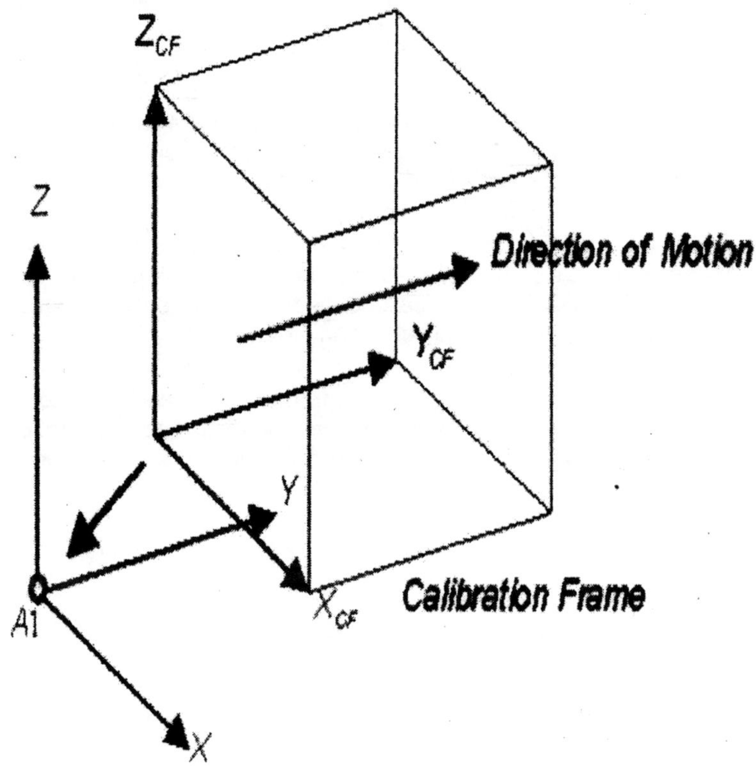

Figure 1

The $X_{CF}Y_{CF}Z_{CF}$ system shown in Figure 1 is the reference frame fixed to the calibration frame while the XYZ system is the new (translated) frame. Marker *A*1 is the additional point. Only the origin of the reference frame moves in this method while the unit vectors of the axes remain intact.

2-Point Method

This method can be used when the vertical axis is aligned properly but the horizontal axes are not (Figure 2). Two additional points are used in this method: *A*1 and *A*2. *A*1 serves as the origin while *A*2 determines the direction of one horizontal axis (the *Y* axis in the example shown in Figure 2). As a result, the *Y* axis of the global reference frame will be aligned with the direction of motion in Figure 2.

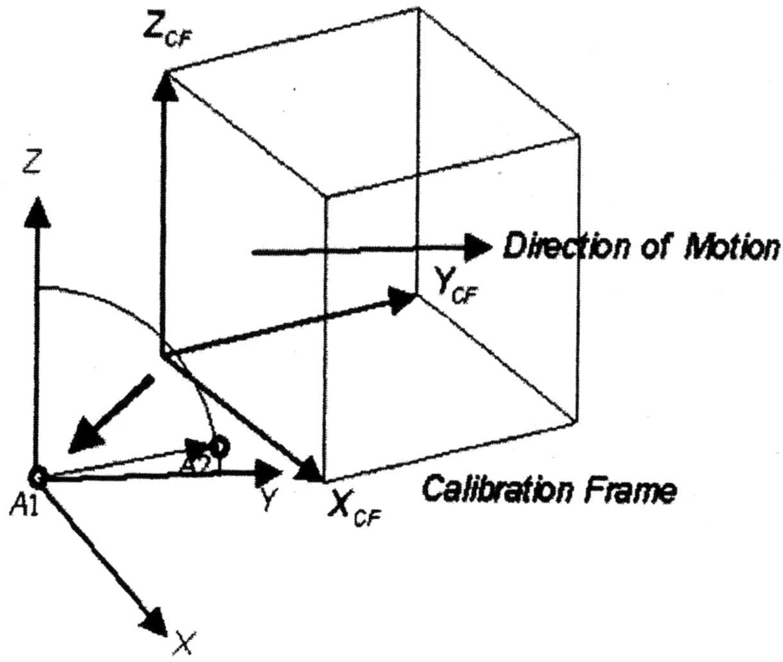

Figure 2

The unit vectors of the new reference frame can be obtained as

$$\mathbf{i} = \frac{\mathbf{A} \times \mathbf{k}}{|\mathbf{A} \times \mathbf{k}|}$$

$$\mathbf{j} = \mathbf{k} \times \mathbf{i} \qquad [1]$$

where **i**, **j**, **k** = the unit vectors of the global reference frame (**k** is known already), and **A** = the vector drawn from *A*1 to *A*2. In other words, *A*2 does not have to be exactly on the *Y* axis. As long as the vector drawn from *A*1.to *A*2 is in the *YZ* plane, both *X* and *Y* axes will be defined correctly. (Remember it was initially assumed that the vertical axis was properly aligned.)

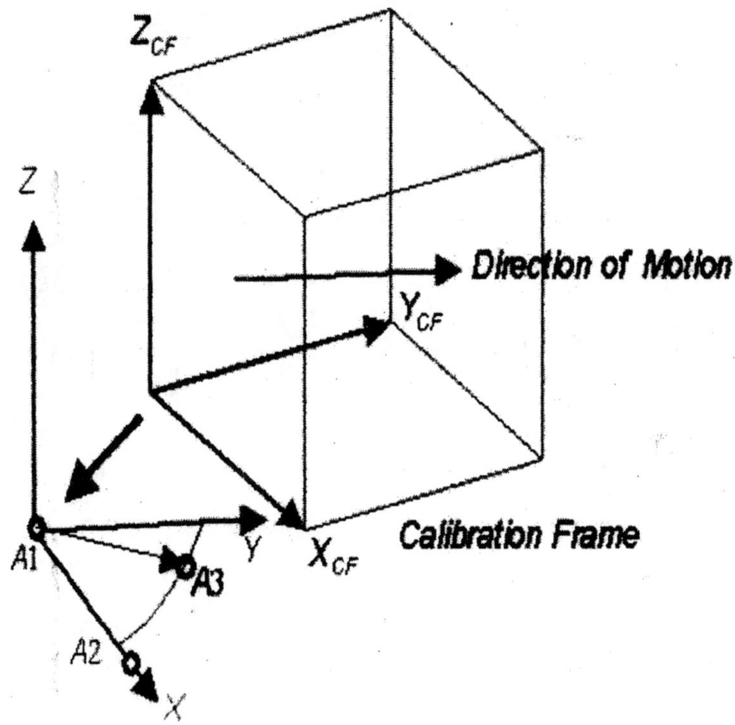

Figure 3

3-Point Method

This method can be used when none of the axes of the reference frame fixed to the calibration frame is aligned properly (Figure 3). Three additional points must be placed on the flat surface: *A*1, *A*2, and *A*3. Two vectors can be defined from the three additional points:

A drawn from *A*1 to *A*2 and **B** drawn from *A*1 to *A*3. **A** accurately defines one horizontal axis (the *X* axis in Figure 3) while **B** serves as the temporary second horizontal axis (the Y axis).

The unit vectors of the new reference frame can be obtained as

$$\mathbf{i} = \frac{\mathbf{A}}{|\mathbf{A}|}$$

$$\mathbf{k} = \frac{\mathbf{i} \times \mathbf{B}}{|\mathbf{i} \times \mathbf{B}|}$$

$$\mathbf{j} = \mathbf{k} \times \mathbf{i} \qquad [2]$$

In other words, the first horizontal axis must be precisely defined by *A*1 and *A*2 but A3 does not have to be on the 2nd horizontal axis.

It will be fine as long as both vectors **A** and **B** are perpendicular to the 3rd axis (the Z axis in Figure 3) thus defines the plane that is perpendicular to the *Z* axis.

The Additional Point Strategies in 2-D Analysis

Two additional point strategies can be used in the 2-D analyses with up to 2 additional points.

No. of Additional Points	Axis Transformation Strategy

1	Translation only
2	1-Axis Rotation + Translation

These are similar to those of the 3-D analysis strategies.

The 1-point method is for translation only.

By placing one additional point in the field, one can move the origin of the global reference frame (translate the reference frame) (Figure 4).

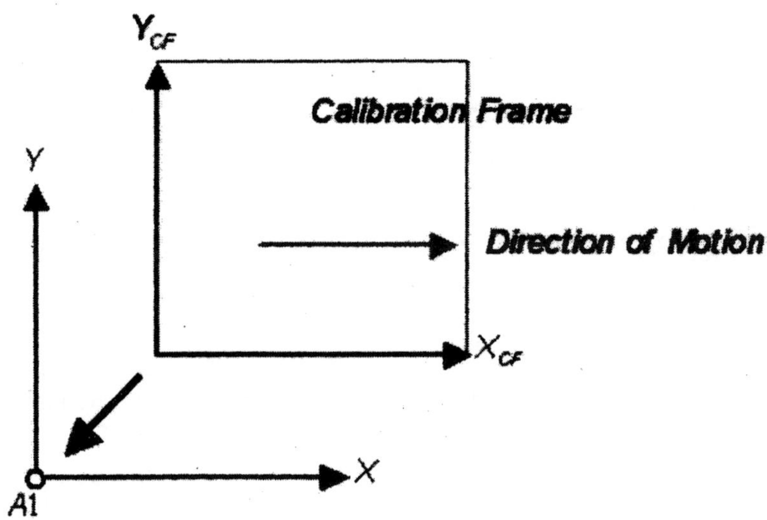

Figure 4

The 2-point method can be used when the axes are not properly aligned with the direction of motion. Two additional points, *A*1 and *A*2 shown in Figure 5, defines one axis (X axis in this example).

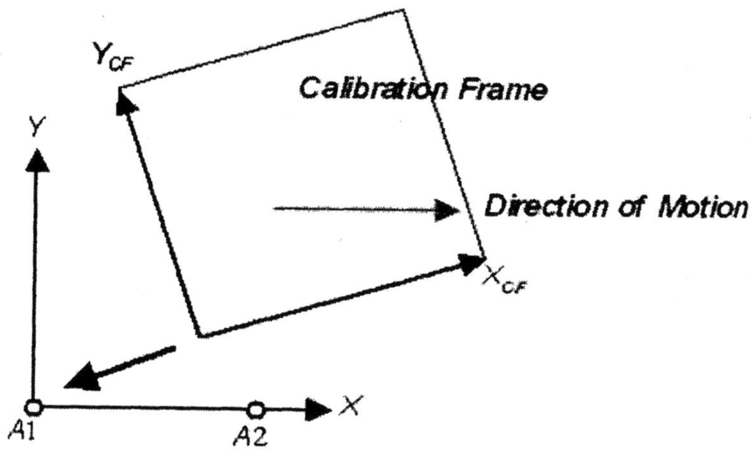

Figure 5

The unit vectors of the new global frame can be obtained as follows:

$$\mathbf{i} = \frac{\mathbf{A}}{|\mathbf{A}|}$$

$$\mathbf{j} = (0,0,1) \times \mathbf{i} \quad [3]$$

where **A** = the vector drawn from *A*1 to *A*2, and **i**, **j** = unit vectors of the global axes. **i**, **j** and **A** are all 3-D vectors with their third components being 0.

Application

The axis alignment based on the additional points is extremely useful when one collects the ground reaction force data in conjunction with motion analysis. In order to combine both data sets for, perhaps, inverse dynamics one must unify the reference frames. Figure 4 illustrates the reference frames involved in this situation.

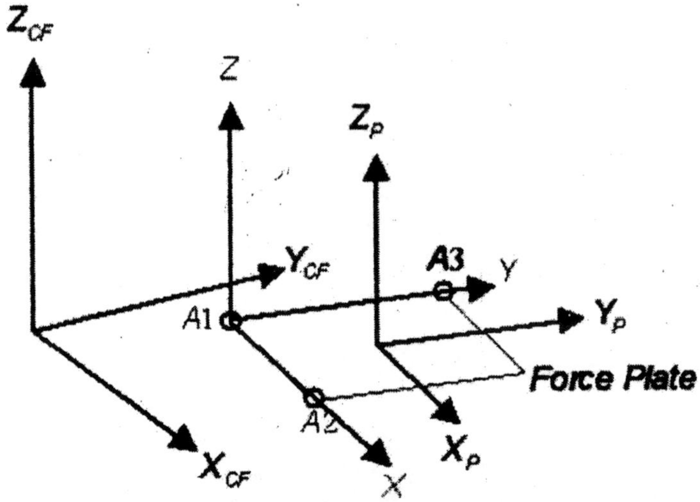

Figure 6

The plate reference frame ($X_P Y_P Z_P$ system in Figure 4) is fixed to the center of the surface of the plate. By using three corners of the plate as additional points, one can define the global reference frame at one corner (*A*1) of the plate. Therefore, the axes of the new global reference frame become parallel to those of the plate reference frame. By translating the force plate reference frame to the global reference frame located at the corner, one can unify the reference frames used in the motion analysis and in the ground reaction force analysis. In reality, one needs to translate the center of pressure data only because the axes of the two systems are already parallel. The dimension of the plate is known, so this should be a simple matter.

Placing markers at the corners of the plate may cause problems in some cases and it is often advantageous to use a set of specially-designed markers for this purpose. Figure 7 shows an example.

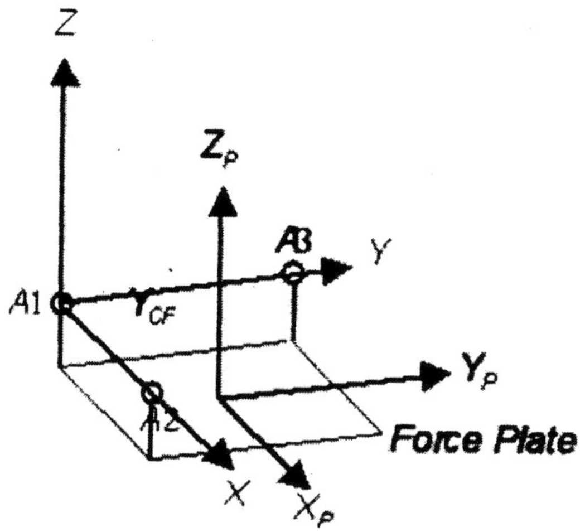

Figure 7

The additional markers in Figure 7 are not on the surface but above the plate. The height of the marker is known so the origin of the reference frame can be easily translated back to the surface of the plate.

The human body can be modeled as a linked-segment system. Here, each segment is regarded as a rigid body and the segments are linked to each other at the joints. But if the focus of the analysis is on the whole body CM kinematics, it is no different from a system of particles. In other words, depending on the analysis focus, one may view the human bocy in different ways.

In many motion analysis systems body modeling is just a pre-step of the marker digitizing or tracking. Although a body model in these systems contain the inertial properties (body segment parameters; BSPs) of the segments, they are often very limited. The typical BSP data allowed in the model are the BSP ratios such as the mass ratios, CM location ratios, and the ROG (radius of gyration) ratios.

In fact, body modeling s much more than a pre-step of marker tracking. It is the process to lay the foundation for the data analysis. It is the process to define the mechanical system. One needs to confine the scope of the mechanical system and to define its nature with a body model. A body model is indeed a collection of all the relevant pieces of information about the body to be analyzed. The main elements of a body model are the points, segments (rigid bodies), segment groups (systems of rigid bodies), and the joints.

The pages included in this section are:

- Point Modeling
- Segment Modeling
- Segment Group Modeling
- Joint Modeling

The body segment parameters (BSPs) refer to the inertial parameters of the body segments, such as mass, CM location and three principal moments of inertia. CM location is used in computing the location of the segmental CM. Segmental masses along with the segmental CM positions are used in computing the CM of the system of rigid bodies such as the whole body. The principal moments of inertia are used in the angular kinetics.

The inertial parameters relate the kinematic quantities to the kinetic quantities. All the kinetic quantities include the inertial properties, mass and moment of inertia (inertia tensor), in the formula. In other words, the accuracy in the kinetic analysis partially depends on the accuracy of the BSPs used.

Investigators generally choose the BSP estimation method from a pool of available estimation methods. Different from the random experimental errors involved in the digitizing and anthropometric measurement, the error from the method of BSP estimation can be systematic. More individualized methods would provide more accurate BSPs. Group-oriented BSP estimation methods may generate inaccurate BSPs for each individual. In other words, individualization of the BSPs to some extent would be necessary.

The issues in this section are:

- BSP Handling Strategies
- BSP Estimation Methods

For geometric inertia models, one has to deal with a group of known geometric shapes. The BSP functions, such as the volume, CM, and volume moments of inertia, are compiled in BSP Equations of the Geometric Shapes.

Group- vs. Individual-Oriented BSP Handling Strategies

The group-oriented approach has been used almost exclusively in the general-purpose motion analysis packages including ***Kwon3D 1.0*** (released in 1991). In other words, the BSP ratios (CM to segment-length ratio, mass to whole body mass ratio, & radius of gyration to segment length ratios) are registered in the model file and applied to all the subjects or trials. Several problems have been encountered in this approach:

The group-oriented approach can not accommodate any foreign object the mass & moments of inertia (MOIs) of which vary from one trial to another, and from one subject to another. In the worst case, one must create a model file for each trial.

The group-oriented approach does not allow individualization of the BSPs since it is based on the BSP ratios.

In order to overcome these problems, one must use an individual-oriented BSP handling strategy. The best way to do this is to separate the BSP data from the body-model file and store them in the so-called BSP files. A BSP file can contain either the group-oriented BSP ratios or the individualized BSP data. In other words, the approach to be used depends on the nature of the BSP file: group-oriented or individual-oriented. The BSP data can be read into the trial file from the specified BSP file.

Several BSP estimation methods are listed under BSP Estimation Methods. The degree of individualization varies from one method to another. See the individual method pages for the details.

Common vs. Trial-Specific BSPs

One problem not completely solved yet with the individual-oriented approach is the trial-specific BSPs. This is mainly due to the use of foreign object segments. When the subject uses tools such as racquet, bat or barbell as a part of the body, these must be included in the model.

For example, if one wants to see the effects of barbell weight on the lifting technique and the weight of the barbell changes from one trial to another, the inertial properties of the barbell, thus, are trial-specific. To accommodate this need, one must create a BSP file for each trial, which is not quite desirable. Here are the solutions:

Store all the common BSPs in the BSP file.

House a BSP editor in the program (at the trial level) to allow editing of the BSP data. Enter the trial-specific BSPs in this editor environment.

Set up the editor to accept both the BSP ratios and the actual BSP data. This will allow the investigator to use the trial-specific BSPs in combination with either the group-oriented or the individual-oriented BSP handling strategy.

The combination of group/individual-oriented strategy and the common/trial-specific BSPs prevents investigators from creating multiple BSP files for the same subject or subject group.

Segment IDs

Separation of the BSP data from the body model causes one minor problem. While reading the BSP data into the trial file from the BSP file, the analysis program must be informed of the types of segments included in the model. The segment name used in the modeling process do not necessarily inform the program of the segment types. One way to nicely solve this problem is to use the segment ID numbers. For example, here is the ID # system used in ***Kwon3D***:

ID #	Description
0	Body part: does not require BSPs
1-12	Reserved human body segments
13-20	User-defined human body segments
21-30	Foreign object segments
31-35	Imaginary segments

ID #	Description
1	Hand
2	Forearm
3	Upperarm
4	Foot
5	Shank
6	Thigh
7	Head
8	Thorax
9	Abdomen
10	Pelvis
11	Thorax-Abdomen
12	Whole Trunk

During the body modeling process, one can specify the segment types by using the ID numbers. The analysis program will then read in the right BSP data from the registered BSP file.

Another important advantage of using the segment ID numbers is the compatibility between the BSP estimation programs and the BSP file. One may use the same ID number system in the BSP estimation programs to secure a complete compatibility among the estimation method, BSP file, and the body model. In other words, the BSP files can be created by the BSP estimation programs, which will then be used by the analysis program.

BSP Estimation Methods

The BSP estimation methods presented here were originally compiled by *Kwon (1993)*. Three groups of BSP estimation methods are included in this page: the cadaver-based (group C), the mass-scanning based (group M) & the geometric models (group G):

Cadaver-Based

- Ratio Method
- Simple Regression Method
- Stepwise Regression Method

- Scaling Method

Mass Scanning-Based

- Ratio Method
- Simple Regression Method
- Prediction Equation Method
- Scaling Method

Geometric Models

- Modified Hanavan (Hanavan-Kwon)
- Modified Yeadon (Yeadon-Kwon)

Three general geometric shapes were used in group G to define the body segments: semi-ellipsoid, elliptical solid and stadium solid. See BSP Equations for the details of the BSP equations of these general geometric shapes, such as the volume, CM location, and the volume moments of inertia.

All methods listed above require a set of anthropometric parameters. See Anthropometric Measurement for the details.

Selection Criteria

The method-selection criteria are: (a) all three principal moments of inertia for each segment should be provided, (b) the BSPs of the sub-trunk segments should be provided, and (c) the BSP estimation process should be relatively simple. The work done by Chandler et al. and Zatsiorsky et al., and the geometric methods were first selected based on the first criterion. Among the geometric methods, the elliptical zone method (Jensen, 1978) and the Hatze model (Hatze, 1980) were dropped based on the third criterion since these methods require either complex data collection and additional equipment, or extensive anthropometric measurement.

In all methods except the modified Yeadon model, the trunk was sectioned at the xyphion and omphalion levels into 3 segments: upper (thorax including neck), middle (abdomen) and lower (pelvis). The CM locations and radius-of-gyration ratios were expressed in % of the hip-to-omphalion height, omphalion-to-xyphion height and the xyphion-to-shoulder height in the lower, middle and upper trunks, respectively. The BSPs of the upper and middle trunks were combined to obtain those of the thorax-abdomen. The modified Yeadon model directly generates the BSPs of the thorax-abdomen.

Mass & MOI Correction

Due to the errors involved in mass estimation, the masses and moments of inertia of the segments must be corrected based on the measured whole body mass:

Estimation of the whole body mass based on the estimated segment masses:

$$M_e = \sum_i m_i(est) \quad [1]$$

Calculation of the density factor from the measured and the estimated whole-body masses:

$$df = \frac{M}{M_e} \quad [2]$$

Correction of the masses and the principal moments of inertia of the segments:

$$\begin{aligned} m_i &= m_i(est) \cdot df \\ I_{xx_i} &= I_{xx_i}(est) \cdot df \\ I_{yy_i} &= I_{yy_i}(est) \cdot df \\ I_{zz_i} &= I_{zz_i}(est) \cdot df \end{aligned} \quad [3]$$

BSP Equations

Three geometric groups commonly used in defining the body segments are semi-ellipsoids, elliptical solids and stadium solids.

The semi-ellipsoid group consists of semi-ellipsoid, ellipsoid of revolution and sphere. The typical members of the elliptical solid group are the elliptical and circular cylinders, the truncated or normal circular and elliptical cones and the general elliptical and circular solids.

The stadium solid group consists of the stadium solids and the stadium cylinders:

Group	Member Geometric Shapes
Semi-Ellipsoid (SE)	Semi-ellipsoid Ellipsoid Ellipsoid of revolution Sphere
Elliptical Solid (ES)	Elliptical solid Truncated circular cone Elliptical Cylinder Elliptical disk (zone) Circular cylinder
Stadium Solid (SS)	Stadium solid Stadium cylinder

For each geometric group, equations for the mass (*m*), center-of-mass (CM) location from the proximal end (g_z), and the three principal moments of inertia (I_{xx}x, I_{yy} & I_{zz}) are provided.

A uniform density of ρ is assumed here. The BSP equations for the stadium solid were adapted and modified from *Yeadon (1990)*.

Basic Integral Functions

Let functions $a(t)$, $b(t)$, $c(t)$ & $d(t)$ be functions of t

$$a(t) \equiv a\sqrt{1-t^2}$$
$$b(t) \equiv b\sqrt{1-t^2}$$
$$c(t) \equiv c\sqrt{1-t^2}$$
$$d(t) \equiv d\sqrt{1-t^2} \quad \textbf{[1]}$$

where a, b, c, $d \geq 0$ and $0 \leq t \leq 1$. Then,

$$\int_0^1 a(t)\cdot b(t)\cdot dt = ab\int_0^1 \left(1-t^2\right)\cdot dt = ab\left[t - \frac{t^3}{3}\right]_0^1 = \frac{2}{3}ab$$

$$\int_0^1 a(t)\cdot b(t)\cdot t\cdot dt = ab\int_0^1 \left(t-t^3\right)\cdot dt = ab\left[\frac{t^2}{2} - \frac{t^4}{4}\right]_0^1 = \frac{1}{4}ab$$

$$\int_0^1 a(t)\cdot b(t)\cdot t^2\cdot dt = ab\int_0^1 \left(1-t^2\right)t^2\cdot dt = ab\int_0^1 \left(t^2-t^4\right)\cdot dt = ab\left[\frac{t^3}{3} - \frac{t^5}{5}\right]_0^1 = \frac{2}{15}ab$$

$$\int_0^1 a(t)\cdot b(t)\cdot c(t)\cdot d(t)\cdot dt = abcd\int_0^1 \left(1-t^2\right)^2\cdot dt = abcd\int_0^1 \left(1-2t^2+t^4\right)\cdot dt$$

$$= abcd\left[t - \frac{2t^3}{3} + \frac{t^5}{5}\right]_0^1 = \frac{8}{15}abcd$$

[2]

Now, let functions $a(t)$, $b(t)$, $c(t)$ & $d(t)$ be

$$a(t) \equiv (a_1 - a_o)t + a_o$$
$$b(t) \equiv (b_1 - b_o)t + b_o$$
$$c(t) \equiv (c_1 - c_o)t + c_o$$
$$d(t) \equiv (d_1 - d_o)t + d_o \quad \textbf{[3]}$$

where, a_o, a_1, b_o, b_1, c_o, c_1, d_o & $d_1 \geq 0$ and $0 \leq t \leq 1$. Then,

$$G_{20}(a,b) \equiv \int_0^1 a(t)\cdot b(t)\cdot dt$$

$$= \int_0^1 \left[F_{22}(a,b)\cdot t^2 + F_{21}(a,b)\cdot t + F_{20}(a,b)\right] dt = \left[\frac{F_{22}(a,b)}{3}t^3 + \frac{F_{21}(a,b)}{2}t^2 + F_{20}(a,b)\cdot t\right]_0^1$$

$$= \frac{F_{22}(a,b)}{3} + \frac{F_{21}(a,b)}{2} + F_{20}(a,b)$$

$$G_{21}(a,b) \equiv \int_0^1 a(t)\cdot b(t)\cdot t\cdot dt$$

$$= \int_0^1 \left[F_{22}(a,b)\cdot t^3 + F_{21}(a,b)\cdot t^2 + F_{20}(a,b)\cdot t\right]\cdot dt = \left[\frac{F_{22}(a,b)}{4}t^4 + \frac{F_{21}(a,b)}{3}t^3 + \frac{F_{20}(a,b)}{2}t^2\right]_0^1$$

$$= \frac{F_{22}(a,b)}{4} + \frac{F_{21}(a,b)}{3} + \frac{F_{20}(a,b)}{2}$$

$$G_{22}(a,b) \equiv \int_0^1 a(t)\cdot b(t)\cdot t^2\cdot dt$$

$$= \int_0^1 \left[F_{22}(a,b)\cdot t^4 + F_{21}(a,b)\cdot t^3 + F_{20}(a,b)\cdot t^2\right]\cdot dt = \left[\frac{F_{22}(a,b)}{5}t^5 + \frac{F_{21}(a,b)}{4}t^4 + \frac{F_{20}(a,b)}{3}t^3\right]_0^1$$

$$= \frac{F_{22}(a,b)}{5} + \frac{F_{21}(a,b)}{4} + \frac{F_{20}(a,b)}{3}$$

$$
\begin{aligned}
G_{40}(a,b,c,d) &\equiv \int_{0}^{1} a(t)\cdot b(t)\cdot c(t)\cdot d(t)\cdot dt \\
&= \int_{0}^{1}\left[F_{44}(a,b,c,d)\cdot t^4 + F_{43}(a,b,c,d)\cdot t^3 + F_{42}(a,b,c,d)\cdot t^2 + F_{41}(a,b,c,d)\cdot t + F_{40}(a,b,c,d)\right]\cdot dt \\
&= \left[\frac{F_{44}(a,b,c,d)}{5}t^5 + \frac{F_{43}(a,b,c,d)}{4}t^4 + \frac{F_{42}(a,b,c,d)}{3}t^3 + \frac{F_{41}(a,b,c,d)}{2}t^2 + F_{40}(a,b,c,d)\cdot t\right]_{0}^{1} \\
&= \frac{F_{44}(a,b,c,d)}{5} + \frac{F_{43}(a,b,c,d)}{4} + \frac{F_{42}(a,b,c,d)}{3} + \frac{F_{41}(a,b,c,d)}{2} + F_{40}(a,b,c,d)
\end{aligned}
$$

[4]

where

$$
\begin{aligned}
F_{22}(a,b) &\equiv (a_1 - a_0)(b_1 - b_0) \\
F_{21}(a,b) &\equiv a_0(b_1 - b_0) + (a_1 - a_0)b_0 \\
F_{20}(a,b) &\equiv a_0 b_0
\end{aligned}
$$

$$
\begin{aligned}
F_{44}(a,b,c,d) &\equiv (a_1 - a_0)(b_1 - b_0)(c_1 - c_0)(d_1 - d_0) \\
F_{43}(a,b,c,d) &\equiv a_0(b_1 - b_0)(c_1 - c_0)(d_1 - d_0) + (a_1 - a_0)b_0(c_1 - c_0)(d_1 - d_0) \\
&\quad + (a_1 - a_0)(b_1 - b_0)c_0(d_1 - d_0) + (a_1 - a_0)(b_1 - b_0)(c_1 - c_0)d_0 \\
F_{42}(a,b,c,d) &\equiv a_0 b_0(c_1 - c_0)(d_1 - d_0) + a_0(b_1 - b_0)c_0(d_1 - d_0) + a_0(b_1 - b_0)(c_1 - c_0)d_0 \\
&\quad + (a_1 - a_0)b_0 c_0(d_1 - d_0) + (a_1 - a_0)b_0(c_1 - c_0)d_0 + (a_1 - a_0)(b_1 - b_0)c_0 d_0 \\
F_{41}(a,b,c,d) &\equiv (a_1 - a_0)b_0 c_0 d_0 + a_0(b_1 - b_0)c_0 d_0 + a_0 b_0(c_1 - c_0)d_0 + a_0 b_0 c_0(d_1 - d_0) \\
F_{40}(a,b,c,d) &\equiv a_0 b_0 c_0 d_0
\end{aligned}
$$

[5]

A set of trigonometric integral functions were also used in deriving the BSP functions:

$$\int_0^{\pi/2} \cos\theta \cdot d\theta = [\sin\theta]_0^{\pi/2} = 1$$

$$\int_0^{\pi/2} \cos^2\theta \; d\theta = \int_0^{\pi/2} \frac{1+\cos 2\theta}{2} \cdot d\theta = \left[\frac{1}{2} - \frac{\sin 2\theta}{4}\right]_0^{\pi/2} = \frac{\pi}{4}$$

$$\int_0^{\pi/2} \cos^3\theta \cdot d\theta = \int_0^1 \left[1 - t^2\right] \cdot dt = \left[t - \frac{t^3}{3}\right]_0^1 = \frac{2}{3}$$

$$\int_0^{\pi/2} \cos^4\theta \cdot d\theta = \frac{1}{4}\int_0^{\pi/2} [1+\cos 2\theta]^2 \cdot d\theta = \frac{1}{4}\int_0^{\pi/2} \left[1 + 2\cos 2\theta + \cos^2 2\theta\right] \cdot d\theta$$

$$= \frac{1}{4}\int_0^{\pi/2} \left[\frac{3}{2} + 2\cos 2\theta + \frac{\cos 4\theta}{2}\right] \cdot d\theta = \frac{1}{4}\left[\frac{3}{2}\theta - \sin 2\theta - \frac{\sin 4\theta}{8}\right]_0^{\pi/2} = \frac{3\pi}{16}$$

$$\int_0^{\pi/2} \sin^4\theta \cdot d\theta = \int_0^{\pi/2} \left[1 - \cos^2\theta\right]^2 \cdot d\theta = \int_0^{\pi/2} \left[1 - 2\cos^2\theta + \cos^4\theta\right] \cdot d\theta = \frac{3\pi}{16}$$

[6]

Elliptical Plate

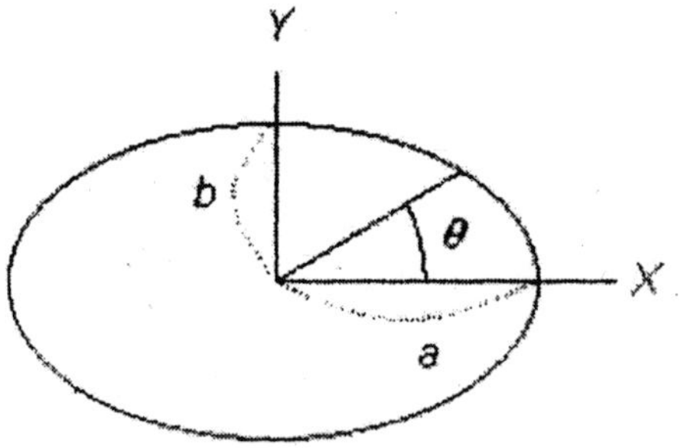

Figure 1

The mass and principal moments of inertia of an elliptical plate (Figure 1) is as follows:

$$m_{ellipse} = 4\rho\int_0^a y \cdot dx = 4\rho b\int_0^a \sqrt{1-\frac{x^2}{a^2}} \cdot dx = 4\rho b\int_0^{\pi/2} \sqrt{1-\sin^2\theta} \cdot d\theta = 4\rho ab\int_0^{\pi/2} \cos^2\theta \cdot d\theta = \pi\rho ab$$

$$J_{xx_{ellipse}} = 4\rho\int_0^a \left[\frac{y^3}{3}\right] \cdot dx = \frac{4}{3}\rho b^3\int_0^a \left[\sqrt{1-\frac{x^2}{a^2}}\right]^3 \cdot dx = \frac{4}{3}\rho b^3\int_0^{\pi/2} \cos^3\theta \cdot [a \cdot \cos\theta \cdot d\theta]$$

$$= \frac{4}{3}\rho ab^3\int_0^{\pi/2} \cos^4\theta \cdot d\theta = \frac{\pi}{4}\rho ab^3$$

$$J_{yy_{ellipse}} = 4\rho\int_0^b \left[\frac{x^3}{3}\right] \cdot dy = -\frac{4}{3}\rho a^3 b\int_{\pi/2}^0 \sin^4\theta \cdot d\theta = \frac{\pi}{4}\rho a^3 b$$

$$J_{zz_{ellipse}} = J_{xx_{ellipse}} + J_{yy_{ellipse}} = \frac{\pi}{4}\rho ab\left[a^2 + b^2\right]$$

[7]

Note that [6] was used in deriving [7].

Semi-Ellipsoid (SE)

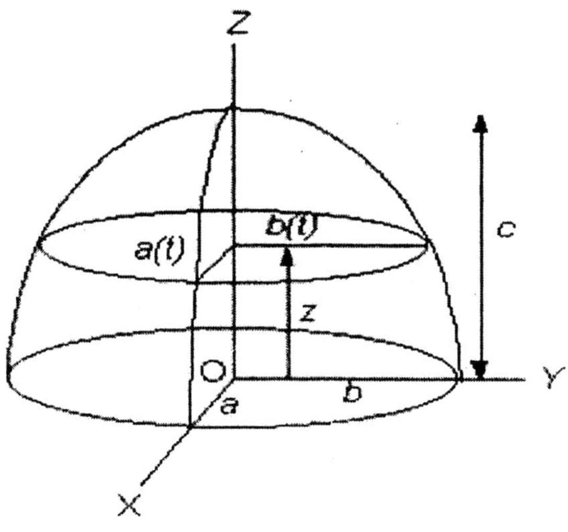

Figure 2

Let z in Figure 2 be a function of t ($0 \leq t \leq 1$):

$$z = ct$$
$$dz = c \cdot dt \qquad \textbf{[8]}$$

Then,

$$m = \int_0^c m_{ellipse}(z) \cdot dz = c\int_0^1 m_{ellipse}(t) \cdot dt = \rho c\int_0^1 a(t) \cdot b(t) \cdot dt = \frac{2\pi}{3}\rho abc$$

$$P_z = \rho\int_0^c m_{ellipse}(z) \cdot z \cdot dz = \rho c^2\int_0^1 m_{ellipse}(t) \cdot t \cdot dt = \pi\rho c^2\int_0^1 a(t) \cdot b(t) \cdot t \cdot dt = \frac{\pi}{4}\rho abc^2$$

$$g_z = \frac{P_z}{m} = \frac{3}{8}c$$

$$I_{zz} = I_z$$

$$= \int_0^c J_{zz_{ellipse}}(z) \cdot dz = c\int_0^1 J_{zz_{ellipse}}(t) \cdot dt = \frac{\pi}{4}\rho c\int_0^1 \left[a(t) \cdot b^3(t) + a^3(t) \cdot b(t)\right] \cdot dt = \frac{\pi}{4}\rho c\left[\frac{8}{15}ab^3 + \frac{8}{15}a^3 b\right]$$

$$= \frac{2\pi}{15}\rho abc\left(a^2 + b^2\right)$$

$$I_X = \int_0^c \left[J_{xx_{ellipse}}(z) + m_{ellipse}(z) \cdot z^2 \right] \cdot dz = \int_0^1 \left[J_{xx_{ellipse}}(t) + m_{ellipse}(t) \cdot c^2 \cdot t^2 \right] c \cdot dt$$

$$= c\int_0^1 J_{xx_{ellipse}}(t) \cdot dt + c^3 \int_0^1 m_{ellipse}(t) \cdot t^2 \cdot dt = \frac{\pi}{4}\rho c \int_0^1 a(t) \cdot b^3(t) \cdot dt + \pi \rho c^3 \int_0^1 a(t) \cdot b(t) \cdot t^2 \cdot dt$$

$$= \frac{2\pi}{15}\rho a b^3 c + \frac{2\pi}{15}\rho a b c^3 = \frac{2\pi}{15}\rho a b c \cdot \left(b^2 + c^2 \right)$$

$$I_{xx} = I_X - m \cdot g_z^{\ 2}$$

$$I_y = \frac{2\pi}{15}\rho a^3 b c + \frac{2\pi}{15}\rho a b c^3 = \frac{2\pi}{15}\rho a b c\left(a^2 + c^2\right)$$

$$I_{yy} = I_y - m \cdot g_z^{\ 2}$$ **[9]**

[2] & [7] were used in deriving [9]. The BSP equations for ellipsoid, ellipsoid of revolution, and sphere can be derived from [9]:

Geometric Shape	Properties
Ellipsoid	$m = 2m_{SE}$, $g_z = 50$ %
Ellipsoid of Revolution	$a = b$, $m = 2m_{SE}$, $g_z = 50$ %
Sphere	$a = b = c$, $m = 2m_{SE}$, $g_z = 50$ %

Elliptical Solid

Let z in Figure 3 be a function of t (where $0 \le t \le 1$):

$$z = Lt$$

$$dz = L \ dt$$ **[10]**

Then,

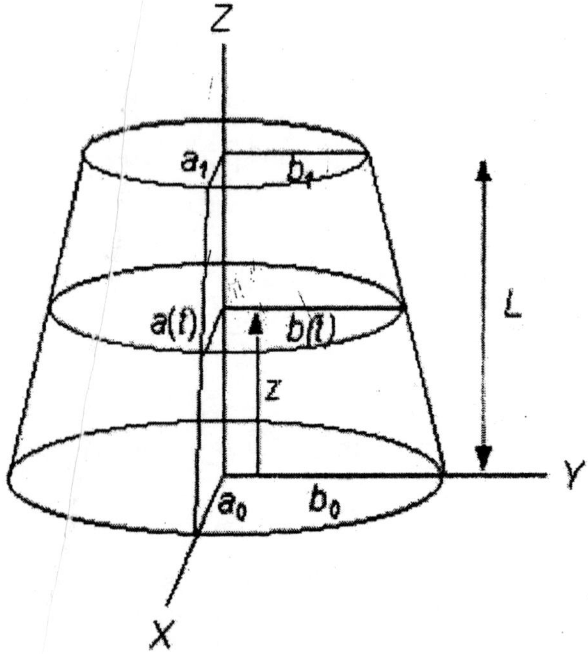

Figure 3

$$m=\int_0^L m_{ellipse}(z)\cdot dz=\pi\rho\int_0^L a(t)\cdot b(t)\cdot L\cdot dt=\pi\rho L\int_0^1 a(t)\cdot b(t)\cdot dt=\pi\rho L\cdot G_{20}(a,b)$$

$$P_z=\int_0^L m_{ellipse}(z)\cdot z\cdot dz=\pi\rho\int_0^L a(t)\cdot b(t)\cdot (Lt)(L\cdot dt)=\pi\rho L^2\int_0^1 a(t)\cdot b(t)\cdot t\cdot dt=\pi\rho L^2\cdot G_{21}(a,b)$$

$$g_z=\frac{P_z}{m}=\frac{G_{21}(a,b)}{G_{20}(a,b)}L$$

$$I_{zz} = I_z$$

$$= \int_0^L J_{zz_{ellipse}}(z) \cdot dz = L\int_0^1 J_{zz_{ellipse}}(t) \cdot dt = \frac{\pi}{4}\rho L\int_0^1 \left[a(t)^3 \cdot b(t) + a(t) \cdot b(t)^3\right] \cdot dt$$

$$= \frac{\pi}{4}\rho L\left[G_{40}(a,a,a,b) + G_{40}(a,b,b,b)\right]$$

$$I_x = \int_0^L \left[J_{xx_{ellipse}}(z) + m(z) \cdot z^2\right] \cdot dz = \frac{\pi}{4}\rho\int_0^L a(z) \cdot b(z)^3 \cdot dz + \pi\rho\int_0^L a(z) \cdot b(z) \cdot z^2 \cdot dz$$

$$= \frac{\pi}{4}\rho L\int_0^1 a(t) \cdot b(t)^3 \cdot dt + \pi\rho L^3\int_0^1 a(t) \cdot b(t) \cdot t^2 \cdot dt = \frac{\pi}{4}\rho L \cdot G_{40}(a,b,b,b) + \pi\rho L^3 \cdot G_{22}(a,b)$$

$$I_{xx} = I_x - m \cdot g_z^{\;2}$$

$$I_y = \int_0^L \left[J_{yy_{ellipse}}(z) + m(z) \cdot z^2\right] \cdot dz = \frac{\pi}{4}\rho L \cdot G_{40}(a,a,a,b) + \pi\rho L^3 \cdot G_{22}(a,b)$$

$$I_{yy} = I_y - m \cdot g_z^{\;2}$$

[11]

direction of the *X* axis is independent from a motion in the direction of the *Y* axis.

3-D Cartesian Coordinates

The 3-D Cartesian coordinate system deals with 3 mutually perpendicular straight lines or axes (Figure 2). Again, one can describe the position of point *P* in terms of three Cartesian coordinates: *x*, *y* & *z*. Starting from the origin, one can reach point *P* by moving in the direction of the *X* axis by *x*, in the direction of the *Y* axis by *y*, and in the direction of the *Z* axis by *z*. The sequence here, again, does not matter.

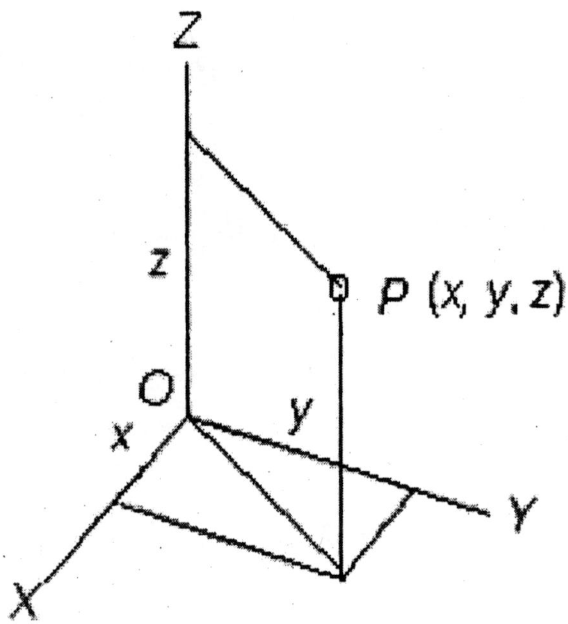

Figure 2

Note in Figure 2 that the *Z* axis is aligned vertically. This is the traditional 3-D Cartesian coordinate system and will be used consistently throughout this website. Those who are accustomed to the *ISB* convention, in which the Y axis is aligned vertically, should switch the axes properly

2-D (Plane) Polar Coordinates

The 2-D polar coordinate system involves the distance from the origin and an azimuth angle. Figure 1 shows the 2-D polar coordinate system, where r is the distance from the origin to point P, and θ is the azimuth angle measured from the horizontal (X) axis in the counterclockwise direction. Thus, the position of point P is described as (r, θ). r & θ are the 2-D polar coordinates.

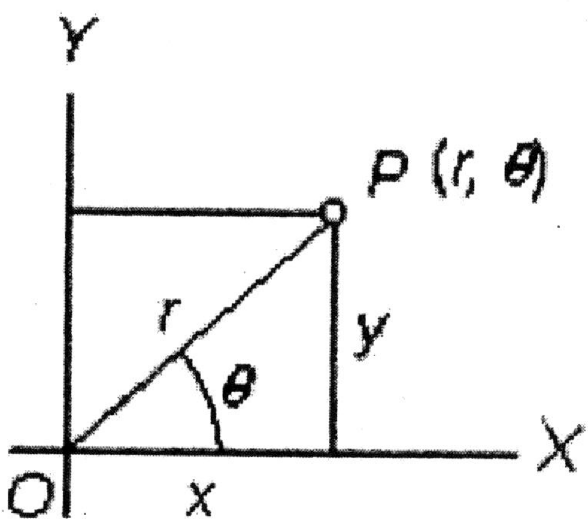

Figure 1

The polar coordinates are useful in describing the human body motion since the essence of the human body motion is the joint motions. The segments undergo rotations about the joint centers and using the azimuth angle (while r = const) in describing the body motion is more efficient than using the Cartesian coordinates. One thing to note here is that ccordinates r & θ are not the same kind.

The relationship between the 2-D Cartesian coordinates and the 2-D polar coordinates can be summarized as

$$r = \sqrt{x^2 + y^2}$$

$$\theta = \begin{cases} \tan^{-1}\left(\dfrac{y}{x}\right) & (x > 0) \\ \tan^{-1}\left(\dfrac{y}{x}\right) + \pi & (x < 0, y > 0) \\ \tan^{-1}\left(\dfrac{y}{x}\right) - \pi & (x < 0, y < 0) \\ \dfrac{\pi}{2} & (x = 0, y > 0) \\ -\dfrac{\pi}{2} & (x = 0, y < 0) \end{cases} \qquad \textbf{[1]}$$

where $-\pi \leq \theta < \pi$. Or

$$x = r \cdot \cos\theta$$
$$y = r \cdot \sin\theta \qquad \textbf{[2]}$$

In some cases, one may use the Cartesian coordinates in the sense of the polar coordinates, as shown on Figure 2.

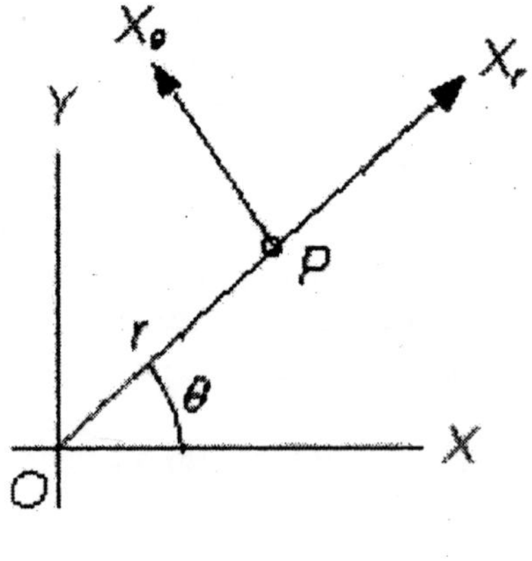

Figure 2

The X_r axis is the radial axis while the X_ϕ axis is the tangential axis. Using the *P*-X_r X_ϕ system (using the Cartesian system in the sense of the polar system) is sometimes more convenient than using the polar coordinate system since it combines the advantages of both systems. Motion in the direction of the X_r axis is the radial motion while that in the direction of the X_ϕ axis reflects the motion due to rotation. One problem here is that the orientation of the X_r & X_ϕ axes changes as point *P* moves.

3-D (Spherical) Polar Coordinates

The 3-D polar coordinate system or the spherical coordinate system involves the distance from the origin and 2 angles (Figure 3).

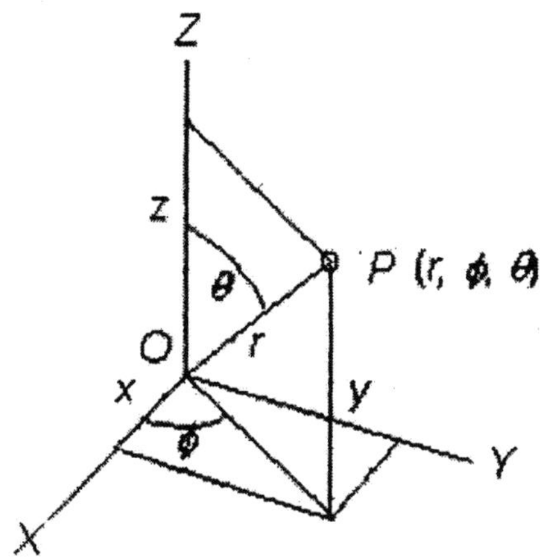

Figure 3

The position of point P is described as (*r*, ϕ, θ), where *r* = the distance from the origin (*O*), ϕ= the horizontal azimuth angle measured on the *XY* plane from the *X* axis in the counterclockwise direction, and θ= the azimuth angle measured from the *Z* axis. Again, the coordinates are not the same kind.

The relationship between the spherical coordinates and the Cartesian coordinates can be summarized as

$$r = \sqrt{x^2 + y^2 + z^2}$$

$$\phi = \begin{cases} \tan^{-1}\left(\frac{y}{x}\right) & (x > 0) \\ \tan^{-1}\left(\frac{y}{x}\right) + \pi & (x < 0, y > 0) \\ \tan^{-1}\left(\frac{y}{x}\right) - \pi & (x < 0, y < 0) \\ \frac{\pi}{2} & (x = 0, y > 0) \\ -\frac{\pi}{2} & (x = 0, y < 0) \end{cases}$$

$$\theta = \begin{cases} \tan^{-1}\left(\frac{\sqrt{x^2 + y^2}}{z}\right) & (z > 0) \\ \tan^{-1}\left(\frac{\sqrt{x^2 + y^2}}{z}\right) + \pi & (z < 0) \\ \frac{\pi}{2} & (z = 0) \end{cases} \qquad [3]$$

where $-\pi \leq \phi < \pi$ and $0 \leq \theta \leq \pi$. Or

$$x = (r \cdot \sin\theta) \cdot \cos\phi = r \cdot \cos\phi \cdot \sin\theta$$
$$y = (r \cdot \sin\theta) \cdot \sin\phi = r \cdot \sin\phi \cdot \sin\theta$$
$$z = r \cdot \cos\theta \qquad [4]$$

Similar to the 2-D moving Cartesian coordinate system shown in Figure 2, one can also define a moving 3-D Cartesian system. See Figure 4. Axis X_r is the radial axis while axes X_ϕ & X_θ shows the normal axes to X_r.

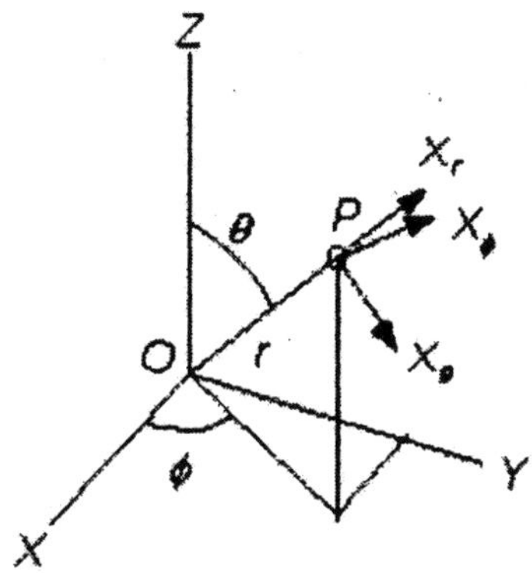

Figure 4

The moving 3-D Cartesian coordinate system shown in Figure 4 is useful in describing the motion of point *P* in terms of the radial motion and the rotations about the origin. Note here that the Cartesian coordinate system shown in Figure 4 is a right-hand system. On the contrary, the Cartesian system normally used in biomechanics or motion analysis is a left-hand system.

The unit vectors (see Vector for the details of the unit vector) of the axes can be described in those of the global reference frame. Let the three unit vectors of system *O-XYZ* be **i**, **j**, and **k**. The unit vectors of system *P*-X_r X_ϕ X_θ ($\mathbf{e}_r$, $\mathbf{e}_\phi$, and $\mathbf{e}_\theta$) are then

$$\mathbf{e}_r = \mathbf{i}\cos\phi\sin\theta + \mathbf{j}\sin\phi\sin\theta + \mathbf{k}\cos\theta$$
$$\mathbf{e}_\phi = -\mathbf{i}\sin\phi + \mathbf{j}\cos\phi$$
$$\mathbf{e}_\theta = \mathbf{i}\cos\phi\cos\theta + \mathbf{j}\sin\phi\cos\theta - \mathbf{k}\sin\theta \quad [5]$$

Most of the mechanical quantities one has to deal with in motion analysis, such as linear & angular position, velocity and acceleration of the markers & segments, are vectors.

Because a vector has both magnitude and direction, one can describe the same vector in several different perspectives, depending on the intention or objective of the analysis. Describing a vector in a particular perspective is in essence equivalent to computing its components based the coordinate system of the particular perspective.

In other words, one can not only describe the same vector in several different perspectives, but also change the perspective from one to another depending on the situation and needs. This changing perspective of describing a vector is called **vector transformation** or **axis transformation**.

The issues covered in this section are:

- Reference Frames
- Transformation Matrix
- Rotation Matrix

One thing to note is the difference between **describing** a vector and **observing** a vector. Observation means one moves with the perspective, and as a result, the outcome is the motion of the body relative to the observer's perspective. The motion (vector) of an object observed in one perspective is different from the same motion observed in another perspective.

For example, to the spectators, a gymnast's airborne maneuver is perceived as a complex motion with both translation of the body CM and rotation (somersault & twist) of the body about its CM. But the same maneuver can be perceived slightly differently by people watching it on TV since the motion of the camera compensates translation of the body CM.

Thus, one can only see the rotation of the body on the screen. Moreover, the gymnast's own perception of the maneuver is very different from those of the spectators and TV watchers. The gymnast only sees the motions of the body parts relative to his/her perspective.

Observation of a vector in a perspective is simply a process of computing the vector relative to the perspective employed. In this process, one can still **describe** the relative vector in different perspectives. See Motion in a Rotating Reference Frame for the details of the quantification of the relative motion.

A reference frame is a particular perspective employed by the analyst to describe and/or observe a motion effectively. There are different types of reference frames. A **fixed frame** is a reference frame that is fixed. A **moving frame** is a reference frame that moves with the body.

A moving reference frame can **translate** and/or **rotate**. When a reference frame is either fixed or moving with a constant velocity, it is an **inertial frame**. An accelerating reference frame is a **non-inertial frame**. A fixed reference frame fixed to the environment, not to the moving subject, and used commonly in describing the motions of different body parts is the **global frame** while all the reference frames fixed to the moving body parts are called the **local frames**.

Among the perspectives presented in Axis Transformation as example, the spectators' perspective is an inertial, fixed, and global frame. The TV watcher's perspective is a moving (translating), non-inertial and local reference frame. The gymnast's perspective is a moving (rotating), non-inertial and local reference frame.

The term "coordinate system" is slightly different from "reference frame". The coordinate system determines the way one describes/observes the motion in each reference frame.

Two types of coordinate systems are commonly used in biomechanics: the **Cartesian system** and the **polar system**. See Coordinate Systems for details of these coordinate systems. One can describe a motion differently in the same perspective depending on the coordinate system employed.

Figure 1 shows examples of different reference frames used to describe the human body motion. One can easily define a local reference frame for each body segment.

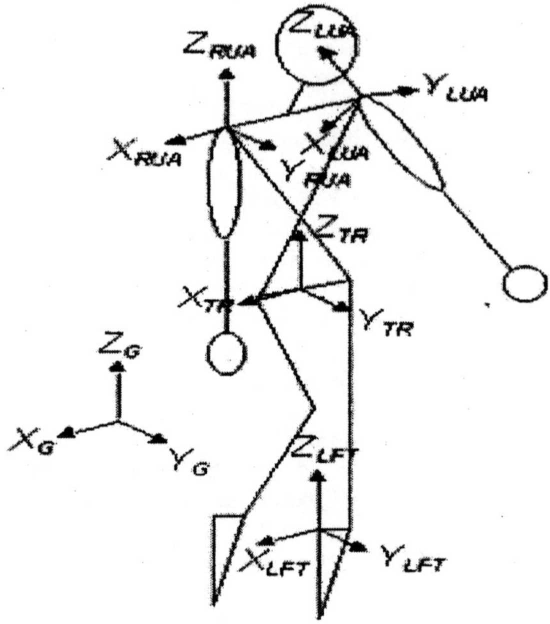

Figure 1

Transformation Matrix

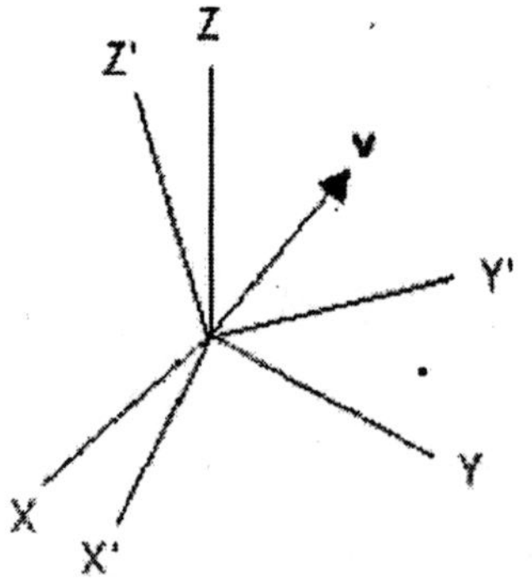

Figure 1

To transform a vector from one reference frame to another is equivalent to changing the perspective of describing the vector from one to another (Figure 1). A transformation alters not the vector, but the components:

$$v'_x = \mathbf{v}\cdot\mathbf{i}' = \left(v_x\mathbf{i} + v_y\mathbf{j} + v_z\mathbf{k}\right)\cdot\mathbf{i}' = v_x\mathbf{i}\cdot\mathbf{i}' + v_y\mathbf{j}\cdot\mathbf{i}' + v_z\mathbf{j}\cdot\mathbf{i}'$$

$$v'_y = \mathbf{v}\cdot\mathbf{j}' = \left(v_x\mathbf{i} + v_y\mathbf{j} + v_z\mathbf{k}\right)\cdot\mathbf{j}' = v_x\mathbf{i}\cdot\mathbf{j}' + v_y\mathbf{j}\cdot\mathbf{j}' + v_z\mathbf{j}\cdot\mathbf{j}'$$

$$v'_z = \mathbf{v}\cdot\mathbf{k}' = \left(v_x\mathbf{i} + v_y\mathbf{j} + v_z\mathbf{k}\right)\cdot\mathbf{k}' = v_x\mathbf{i}\cdot\mathbf{k}' + v_y\mathbf{j}\cdot\mathbf{k}' + v_z\mathbf{j}\cdot\mathbf{k}'$$

$$\begin{bmatrix} v'_x \\ v'_y \\ v'_z \end{bmatrix} = \begin{bmatrix} \mathbf{i}\cdot\mathbf{i}' & \mathbf{j}\cdot\mathbf{i}' & \mathbf{k}\cdot\mathbf{i}' \\ \mathbf{i}\cdot\mathbf{j}' & \mathbf{j}\cdot\mathbf{j}' & \mathbf{k}\cdot\mathbf{j}' \\ \mathbf{i}\cdot\mathbf{k}' & \mathbf{j}\cdot\mathbf{k}' & \mathbf{k}\cdot\mathbf{k}' \end{bmatrix} \begin{bmatrix} v_x \\ v_y \\ v_z \end{bmatrix}$$

[1]

where **i**, **j** & **k** = the unit vectors of the *XYZ* system, and **i**', **j**' & **k**' = the unit vectors of the *X'Y'Z'* system. Therefore, the **transformation matrix** from the global reference frame (frame *G*) to a particular local reference frame (frame *L*) can be written as

$$\begin{bmatrix} v'_x \\ v'_y \\ v'_z \end{bmatrix} = \mathbf{T}_{L/G} \cdot \begin{bmatrix} v_x \\ v_y \\ v_z \end{bmatrix}$$

$$\mathbf{T}_{L/G} = \begin{bmatrix} \mathbf{i}\cdot\mathbf{i}' & \mathbf{j}\cdot\mathbf{i}' & \mathbf{k}\cdot\mathbf{i}' \\ \mathbf{i}\cdot\mathbf{j}' & \mathbf{j}\cdot\mathbf{j}' & \mathbf{k}\cdot\mathbf{j}' \\ \mathbf{i}\cdot\mathbf{k}' & \mathbf{j}\cdot\mathbf{k}' & \mathbf{k}\cdot\mathbf{k}' \end{bmatrix} \quad \textbf{[2]}$$

The local reference frame is typically fixed to a segment or a body part.

Similarly, $\mathbf{T}_{G/L}$, the **inverse transformation matrix** of $\mathbf{T}_{L/G}$, can also be derived as

$$\mathrm{T}_{G/L} = \begin{bmatrix} \mathbf{i}\cdot\mathbf{i}' & \mathbf{i}\cdot\mathbf{j}' & \mathbf{i}\cdot\mathbf{k}' \\ \mathbf{j}\cdot\mathbf{i}' & \mathbf{j}\cdot\mathbf{j}' & \mathbf{j}\cdot\mathbf{k}' \\ \mathbf{k}\cdot\mathbf{i}' & \mathbf{k}\cdot\mathbf{j}' & \mathbf{k}\cdot\mathbf{k}' \end{bmatrix} \quad \textbf{[3]}$$

In other words, a series of transformation is equivalent to a single transformation directly from the originating frame to the destination frame (*A* to *Z* in [8]). In a sense, it is similar to the arithmetic multiplication of the frame subscripts:

$$Z/A = (Z/Y)\cdot(Y/X)\cdots(B/A)\cdot(A/G) \quad \textbf{[9]}$$

Similarly, the transformation matrix from one local reference frame (*A*) to another (*B*) can be easily obtained through cascading of the transformation matrices:

$$\mathbf{T}_{B/A} = \mathbf{T}_{B/G}\cdot\mathbf{T}_{G/A} = \mathbf{T}_{B/G}\cdot\mathbf{T}_{A/G}^{-1} = \mathbf{T}_{B/G}\cdot\mathbf{T}_{A/G}^{t} \quad \textbf{[10]}$$

Once the transformation matrices from the global reference frame to the local reference frames are known, computation of the transformation matrices among the local reference frames is simply a matter of transposition and multiplication of the transformation matrices.

Translation of the Origin

So far we only have dealt with the rotation of the reference frame. This is normally sufficient in working with free vectors such as velocity, force, etc. But it matters when one deals with the position vectors because positions are described by the arrow drawn from the origin of the reference frame and different frames may have different origins. In other words, when one transforms a position vector from one reference frame to another, the translation of the frame origin must be taken into accounts as well:

$$\begin{bmatrix} x^{(B)} \\ y^{(B)} \\ z^{(B)} \end{bmatrix} = \mathbf{T}_{B/A} \begin{bmatrix} x^{(A)} \\ y^{(A)} \\ z^{(A)} \end{bmatrix} + \begin{bmatrix} t_x^{(B)} \\ t_y^{(B)} \\ t_z^{(B)} \end{bmatrix} \quad \textbf{[11]}$$

or

$$\begin{bmatrix} x^{(B)} \\ y^{(B)} \\ z^{(B)} \end{bmatrix} = \mathbf{T}_{B/A} \cdot \begin{bmatrix} x^{(A)} + t_x^{(A)} \\ y^{(A)} + t_y^{(A)} \\ z^{(A)} + t_z^{(A)} \end{bmatrix} \quad [12]$$

where $(t_x, t_y, t_z)^t$ = the translation matrix. [11] can be used when the translation vector is described in the destination frame coordinates. [12] is for the case where the translation vector is described in the originating frame coordinates.

An alternative from to [11] is

$$\begin{bmatrix} x^{(B)} \\ y^{(B)} \\ z^{(B)} \\ 1 \end{bmatrix} = \left[\begin{array}{ccc|c} & & & t_x^{(B)} \\ & \mathbf{T}_{B/A} & & t_y^{(B)} \\ & & & t_z^{(B)} \\ \hline 0 & 0 & 0 & 1 \end{array}\right] \begin{bmatrix} x^{(A)} \\ y^{(A)} \\ z^{(A)} \\ 1 \end{bmatrix} \quad [13]$$

where $\mathbf{T}_{B/A}$ = the 3x3 transformation matrix from frame *A* to frame *B*. The advantage of [13] is that one can eliminate matrix addition in [11] so that put both the rotation and the translation in a single 4x4 transformation matrix. But it theoretically takes longer computer time due to additional computations.

Axis Rotation Matrices

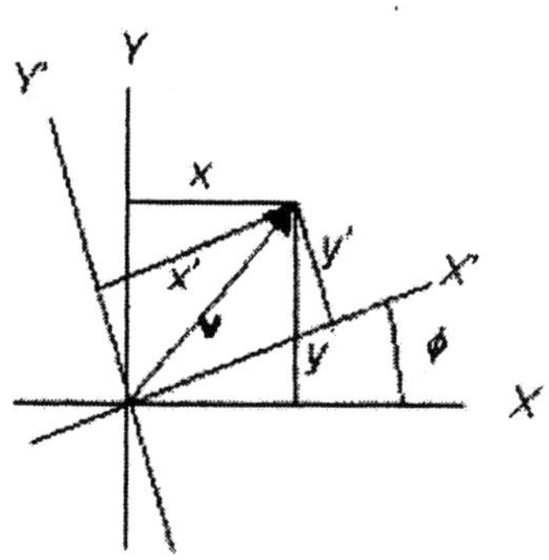

Figure 1

The components of a free vector change as the perspective (reference frame) changes. Figure 1 shows two different reference frames: the *XY* system and the *X'Y'* system. Vector **v** in Figure 1 can be expressed as (*x*, *y*) in the *XY* system, or (*x'*, *y'*) in the *X'Y'* system. The relationships between *x* & *y* and *x'* & *y'* can be obtained from the geometric relationships:

$$x' = x \cdot \cos\phi + y \cdot \sin\phi$$
$$y' = y \cdot \cos\phi - x \cdot \sin\phi$$

$$\begin{bmatrix} x' \\ y' \end{bmatrix} = \begin{bmatrix} \cos\phi & \sin\phi \\ -\sin\phi & \cos\phi \end{bmatrix} \begin{bmatrix} x \\ y \end{bmatrix} \qquad [1]$$

Expanding [1] to 3 dimensions:

$$x' = x \cdot \cos\phi + y \cdot \sin\phi$$
$$y' = y \cdot \cos\phi - x \cdot \sin\phi$$
$$z' = z$$

$$\begin{bmatrix} x' \\ y' \\ z' \end{bmatrix} = \begin{bmatrix} \cos\phi & \sin\phi & 0 \\ -\sin\phi & \cos\phi & 0 \\ 0 & 0 & 1 \end{bmatrix} \begin{bmatrix} x \\ y \\ z \end{bmatrix}$$

$$\mathbf{R}_z(\phi) = \begin{bmatrix} \cos\phi & \sin\phi & 0 \\ -\sin\phi & \cos\phi & 0 \\ 0 & 0 & 1 \end{bmatrix} \qquad [2]$$

[2] is the axis rotation matrix for a rotation about the *Z* axis. Applying the same method to the rotations about the X and the Y axis, respectively:

$$\begin{bmatrix} x' \\ y' \\ z' \end{bmatrix} = \begin{bmatrix} 1 & 0 & 0 \\ 0 & \cos\phi & \sin\phi \\ 0 & -\sin\phi & \cos\phi \end{bmatrix} \begin{bmatrix} x \\ y \\ z \end{bmatrix}$$

$$\mathbf{R}_x(\phi) = \begin{bmatrix} 1 & 0 & 0 \\ 0 & \cos\phi & \sin\phi \\ 0 & -\sin\phi & \cos\phi \end{bmatrix} \quad [3]$$

$$\begin{bmatrix} x' \\ y' \\ z' \end{bmatrix} = \begin{bmatrix} \cos\phi & 0 & -\sin\phi \\ 0 & 1 & 0 \\ \sin\phi & 0 & \cos\phi \end{bmatrix} \begin{bmatrix} x \\ y \\ z \end{bmatrix}$$

$$\mathbf{R}_y(\phi) = \begin{bmatrix} \cos\phi & 0 & -\sin\phi \\ 0 & 1 & 0 \\ \sin\phi & 0 & \cos\phi \end{bmatrix} \quad [4]$$

These matrices for the axis rotations about particular coordinate axes are essential in developing the concept of the **Eulerian/Cardanian angles**. The rotation matrices fulfill the requirements of the transformation matrix. See Transformation Matrix for the details of the requirements.

Axis Rotation vs. Vector Rotation

Figure 2 shows a situation slightly different from that in Figure 1. This time, the vector rather than the axes was rotated about the Z axis by ϕ. This is called the **vector rotation**. In other words, vector $\mathbf{v}_1$ was rotated to $\mathbf{v}_2$ by angle ϕ.

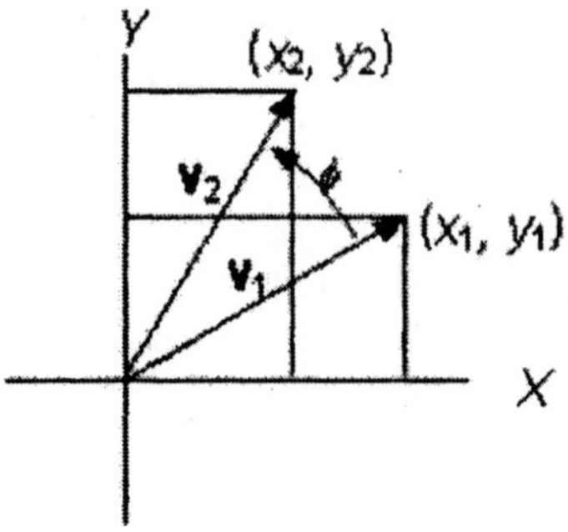

Figure 2

Again, one can obtain the following relationships:

$$x_2 = x_1 \cdot \cos\phi - y_1 \cdot \sin\phi$$
$$y_2 = y_1 \cdot \cos\phi + x_1 \cdot \sin\phi$$

$$\begin{bmatrix} x_2 \\ y_2 \end{bmatrix} = \begin{bmatrix} \cos\phi & -\sin\phi \\ \sin\phi & \cos\phi \end{bmatrix} \begin{bmatrix} x_1 \\ y_1 \end{bmatrix}$$

[5]

since

$$\begin{aligned} x_1 &= r \cdot \cos\alpha \\ y_1 &= r \cdot \sin\alpha \\ x_2 &= r \cdot \cos(\alpha + \phi) = r \cdot (\cos\alpha \cdot \cos\phi - \sin\alpha \cdot \sin\phi) \\ &= x_1 \cdot \cos\phi - y_1 \cdot \sin\phi \\ y_2 &= r \cdot \sin(\alpha + \phi) = r \cdot (\sin\alpha \cdot \cos\phi + \cos\alpha \cdot \sin\phi) \\ &= y_1 \cdot \cos\phi + x_1 \cdot \sin\phi \end{aligned}$$ **[6]**

where r = length of the vector, and α = the angle $\mathbf{v}_1$ makes with the X axis.

Expanding [5] to 3-dimension:

$$x_2 = x_1 \cdot \cos\phi - y_1 \cdot \sin\phi$$
$$y_2 = y_1 \cdot \cos\phi + x_1 \cdot \sin\phi$$
$$z_2 = z_1$$

$$\begin{bmatrix} x_2 \\ y_2 \\ z_2 \end{bmatrix} = \begin{bmatrix} \cos\phi & -\sin\phi & 0 \\ \sin\phi & \cos\phi & 0 \\ 0 & 0 & 1 \end{bmatrix} \begin{bmatrix} x_1 \\ y_1 \\ z_1 \end{bmatrix}$$

$$\mathbf{R}'_z(\phi) = \begin{bmatrix} \cos\phi & -\sin\phi & 0 \\ \sin\phi & \cos\phi & 0 \\ 0 & 0 & 1 \end{bmatrix} \qquad \textbf{[7]}$$

Similarly,

$$\begin{bmatrix} x_2 \\ y_2 \\ z_2 \end{bmatrix} = \begin{bmatrix} 1 & 0 & 0 \\ 0 & \cos\phi & -\sin\phi \\ 0 & \sin\phi & \cos\phi \end{bmatrix} \begin{bmatrix} x_1 \\ y_1 \\ z_1 \end{bmatrix}$$

$$\mathbf{R}'_x(\phi) = \begin{bmatrix} 1 & 0 & 0 \\ 0 & \cos\phi & -\sin\phi \\ 0 & \sin\phi & \cos\phi \end{bmatrix} \qquad \textbf{[8]}$$

and

$$\begin{bmatrix} x_2 \\ y_2 \\ z_2 \end{bmatrix} = \begin{bmatrix} \cos\phi & 0 & \sin\phi \\ 0 & 1 & 0 \\ -\sin\phi & 0 & \cos\phi \end{bmatrix} \begin{bmatrix} x_1 \\ y_1 \\ z_1 \end{bmatrix}$$

$$\mathbf{R}'_y(\phi) = \begin{bmatrix} \cos\phi & 0 & \sin\phi \\ 0 & 1 & 0 \\ -\sin\phi & 0 & \cos\phi \end{bmatrix} \qquad [9]$$

From **[2]** - **[4]** and **[7]** - **[9]**:

$$\mathbf{R}'_x(\phi) = \mathbf{R}_x(-\phi)$$
$$\mathbf{R}'_y(\phi) = \mathbf{R}_y(-\phi)$$
$$\mathbf{R}'_z(\phi) = \mathbf{R}_z(-\phi) \qquad [10]$$

Vector rotation is equivalent to the axis rotation in the opposite direction. One should not be confused by the axis rotation and the vector rotation.

n vector transformation, the axis rotation matrices should be used instead of the vector rotation matrices because vector transformation means change in the perspective.

In motion analysis, investigators generally rely on an inertial reference frame to describe different mechanical quantities.

The typical outcome of a general-purpose motion analysis package includes the position, velocity & acceleration of the joints and the CMs, the angular velocity & acceleration of the segments, and the joint angles & their time-derivatives basically expressed in terms of the inertial reference frame.

One can always express the equations of motion for a system in an inertial reference frame. But there are several occasions where it is more advantageous to use some non-inertial reference frames.

Non-inertial frames allow the investigators to simplify the equations of motion significantly. Using non-inertial frames and subsequently describing different motion quantities in the non-inertial frames can enrich the analysis to a great extent.

The human body consists of several [rigid] segments inter-linked to each other. Motion of a body segment is characterized by the translation of the segment's CM and the rotation about its CM.

One can describe the motion of a distal segment in relation to that of a proximal segment. In this process, one easily encounters a rotating reference frame.

This section explains how to deal with a rotating reference frame to express the motions of equation effectively. The main issues here are:

Displacement Due to an Infinitesimal Rotation

Figure 1 shows the displacement of point *P* due to angular velocity ω. The displacement due to a small amount of rotation *($d\theta$) is denoted as* dr in the figure.

During the rotation point *P* follows a circular path the center of which is located at point *Q*. The radius of this circular path can be described as

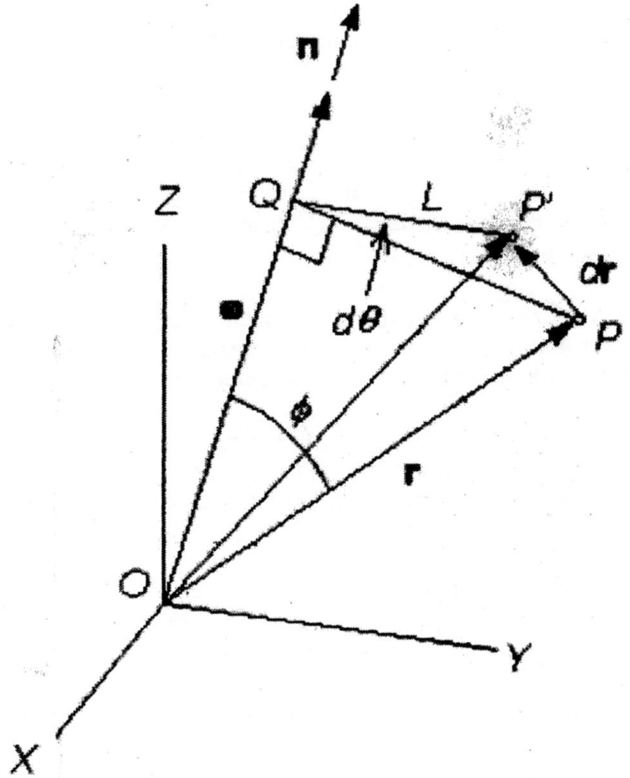

Figure 1

$$L = r \cdot \sin\phi = |\mathbf{n} \times \mathbf{r}| \quad [1]$$

where **n** = the unit vector of angular velocity $\boldsymbol{\omega}$. For a small $d\theta$, the displacement vector is perpendicular to both vectors **n** and **r**, thus,

$$\mathbf{u} = \frac{\mathbf{n} \times \mathbf{r}}{|\mathbf{n} \times \mathbf{r}|} \quad [2]$$

where **u** = the unit vector of displacement vector $d\mathbf{r}$. The length of displacement vector $d\mathbf{r}$ is equal to the length of the arc confined by points *P* and *P'*:

$$dr = L \cdot d\theta \quad [3]$$

Therefore, the displacement vector can be expressed as

$$\begin{aligned} d\mathbf{r} &= dr \cdot \mathbf{u} \\ &= |\mathbf{n} \times \mathbf{r}| \cdot d\theta \frac{\mathbf{n} \times \mathbf{r}}{|\mathbf{n} \times \mathbf{r}|} \\ &= (\mathbf{n} \cdot d\theta) \times \mathbf{r} \\ &= d\boldsymbol{\theta} \times \mathbf{r} \end{aligned} \quad [4]$$

where $d\theta$ = the angular displacement vector. In other words, the displacement due to rotation about an axis of rotation is equal to the cross product of the angular displacement vector and the position vector.

Rotating Reference Frame

Now, let's consider a slightly more complex situation. Figure 2 shows a rotating reference frame, the *X'Y'Z'* system, which rotates at an angular velocity of $\boldsymbol{\omega}$. The inertial reference frame, the *XYZ* system, and the rotating frame share the origin together.

The displacement of point *P* to *P'* is denoted as $d\mathbf{r}$ in the figure. Displacement vector $d\mathbf{r}$ can be split into two elements:

$d\mathbf{r}_R$ and $d\mathbf{r}'$. Vector $d\mathbf{r}_R$ is the displacement due to the rotation of the point with the rotating frame while $d\mathbf{r}'$ is the remainder of the displacement. Thus,

and [12] can be further reduced to

$$\begin{aligned}\frac{d\mathbf{H}}{dt} &= \boldsymbol{\omega}\times\mathbf{H}+\left[\frac{d\mathbf{H}}{dt}\right]_{rot}\\ &= \boldsymbol{\omega}\times\mathbf{H}+\left[\frac{d\mathbf{I}_{CM}}{dt}\boldsymbol{\omega}\right]_{rot}+\left[\mathbf{I}_{CM}\frac{d\boldsymbol{\omega}}{dt}\right]_{rot}\\ &= \boldsymbol{\omega}\times\mathbf{H}+\mathbf{I}_{CM}\left[\frac{d\boldsymbol{\omega}}{dt}\right]_{rot}\\ &= \boldsymbol{\omega}\times\mathbf{H}+\mathbf{I}_{CM}\boldsymbol{\alpha}_r \qquad [13]\end{aligned}$$

since the inertia tensor observed in the rotating frame ($\mathbf{I}_{CM}$) does not change as the body rotates. α_r shown in [13] is the angular acceleration of the body **relative to the rotating frame**. Applying [9] to angular velocity:

$$\begin{aligned}\boldsymbol{\alpha} = \frac{d\boldsymbol{\omega}}{dt} &= \boldsymbol{\omega}\times\boldsymbol{\omega}+\left[\frac{d\boldsymbol{\omega}}{dt}\right]_{rot}\\ &= \left[\frac{d\boldsymbol{\omega}}{dt}\right]_{rot} = \boldsymbol{\alpha}_r \qquad [14]\end{aligned}$$

that is, the angular acceleration observed in the fixed frame is equal to that observed in the rotating frame of the body. Substituting [14] into [13], one can obtain

$$\frac{d\mathbf{H}}{dt} = \boldsymbol{\omega}\times\mathbf{H}+\mathbf{I}_{CM}\boldsymbol{\alpha} \qquad [15]$$

Assuming the axes of the rotating reference frame fixed to the body are principal axes, from [2] of Principal Axes, [15] reduces to

$$\mathbf{T} = \dot{\mathbf{H}} = \begin{bmatrix} 0 & -\omega_z & \omega_y \\ \omega_z & 0 & -\omega_x \\ -\omega_y & \omega_x & 0 \end{bmatrix} \begin{bmatrix} I_{xx}\omega_x \\ I_{yy}\omega_y \\ I_{zz}\omega_z \end{bmatrix} + \begin{bmatrix} I_{xx}\alpha_x \\ I_{yy}\alpha_y \\ I_{zz}\alpha_z \end{bmatrix}$$

$$\begin{bmatrix} T_x \\ T_y \\ T_z \end{bmatrix} = \begin{bmatrix} (I_{zz} - I_{yy})\omega_y\omega_z + I_{xx}\alpha_x \\ (I_{xx} - I_{zz})\omega_z\omega_x + I_{yy}\alpha_y \\ (I_{yy} - I_{xx})\omega_x\omega_y + I_{zz}\alpha_z \end{bmatrix} \qquad [16]$$

[16] is the so-called **Euler's equations** for the motion of a rigid body.

Acceleration of a Particle in a Moving Reference Frame

The *XYZ* system shown in Figure 1 is an inertial reference frame while the *X'Y'Z'* frame is a moving (translation + rotation) reference frame. The position of point *P* in the figure can be expressed in terms of these two reference frames:

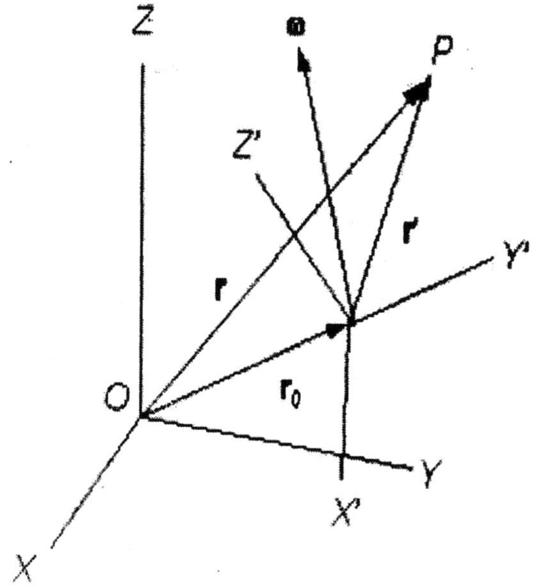

Figure 1

$$\mathbf{r} = \mathbf{r}_o + \mathbf{r}' \quad [1]$$

where $\mathbf{r}_o$ = the position of the origin of the rotating frame, and $\mathbf{r}'$ = the position of *P* relative to the origin of the moving frame.

From [1] and [6] of Rotating Reference Frame, the displacement of point *P* can then be expressed as

$$\begin{aligned} d\mathbf{r} &= d\mathbf{r}_0 + d\mathbf{r}' \\ &= d\mathbf{r}_0 + d\boldsymbol{\theta} \times \mathbf{r}' + [d\mathbf{r}']_{rot} \end{aligned} \quad [2]$$

where $d\mathbf{r}_o$ = the displacement due to translation of the origin of the rotating frame, $d\mathbf{r}'$ = the displacement of point *P* relative to the origin of the rotating frame, $d\theta \times \mathbf{r}'$ = the displacement due to rotation of the moving frame, and $(d\mathbf{r}')_{rot}$ = the displacement of point *P* **observed** in the rotating frame (or the displacement of *P* **relative to the moving frame**).

From [2], the velocity of point *P* can be expressed as

$$\begin{aligned} \mathbf{v} &= \frac{d\mathbf{r}}{dt} = \frac{d\mathbf{r}_0}{dt} + \frac{d\boldsymbol{\theta}}{dt} \times \mathbf{r}' + \left[\frac{d\mathbf{r}'}{dt}\right]_{rot} \\ &= \frac{d\mathbf{r}_0}{dt} + \boldsymbol{\omega} \times \mathbf{r}' + \left[\frac{d\mathbf{r}'}{dt}\right]_{rot} \\ &= \mathbf{v}_0 + \boldsymbol{\omega} \times \mathbf{r}' + \mathbf{v}'_r \end{aligned} \quad [3]$$

where $\mathbf{v}'_r$ = the velocity of point *P* relative to the moving reference frame. Thus, the velocity of point *P* relative to the origin of the moving reference frame can be divided into the velocity due to rotation of the frame and the velocity **observed** in the rotating frame.

Acceleration of point *P* can then be obtained similarly:

$$
\begin{aligned}
\mathbf{a} &= \frac{d\mathbf{v}}{dt} \\
&= \frac{d\mathbf{v}_0}{dt} + \frac{d(\boldsymbol{\omega} \times \mathbf{r}')}{dt} + \frac{d\mathbf{v}'_r}{dt} \\
&= \mathbf{a}_0 + \frac{d\boldsymbol{\omega}}{dt} \times \mathbf{r}' + \boldsymbol{\omega} \times \frac{d\mathbf{r}'}{dt} + \frac{d\mathbf{v}'_r}{dt} \\
&= \mathbf{a}_0 + \dot{\boldsymbol{\omega}} \times \mathbf{r}' + \boldsymbol{\omega} \times \left(\boldsymbol{\omega} \times \mathbf{r}' + \left[\frac{d\mathbf{r}'}{dt} \right]_{rot} \right) + \boldsymbol{\omega} \times \mathbf{v}'_r + \left[\frac{d\mathbf{v}'_r}{dt} \right]_{rot} \\
&= \mathbf{a}_0 + \dot{\boldsymbol{\omega}} \times \mathbf{r}' + \boldsymbol{\omega} \times (\boldsymbol{\omega} \times \mathbf{r}') + \boldsymbol{\omega} \times \mathbf{v}'_r + \boldsymbol{\omega} \times \mathbf{v}'_r + \mathbf{a}'_r \\
&= \mathbf{a}_0 + \dot{\boldsymbol{\omega}} \times \mathbf{r}' + \boldsymbol{\omega} \times (\boldsymbol{\omega} \times \mathbf{r}') + 2\boldsymbol{\omega} \times \mathbf{v}'_r + \mathbf{a}'_r
\end{aligned}
\qquad [4]
$$

where $\mathbf{a}$ = the acceleration of point P, $\mathbf{a}_o$ = the acceleration of the origin of the moving frame, and $\mathbf{a}'_r$ = the acceleration of point P relative to the moving frame. Note here that all vectors involved in the velocity equation shown in [3] are subject to derivation and [9] of Rotating Reference Frame was applied to all cases. [14] of Rotating Reference Frame shows that the time-derivative of the angular velocity vector is not affected by the rotation of the moving frame. As a result, the acceleration of point P shows 5 different terms.

Centripetal Acceleration

The 1st & the 2nd terms in [4] are the results of the translational and rotational acceleration of the moving reference frame, respectively. The 3rd term, $\omega \times (\omega \times \mathbf{r}')$, is due to the rotation of the moving frame and, as shown in Figure 2, this vector heads toward the center of rotation (point C). This acceleration is called the **centripetal acceleration**. The 4th term is due to the motion of the point within the moving frame and is called the **Coriolis acceleration**. The last term is due to the acceleration of the point within the moving reference frame.

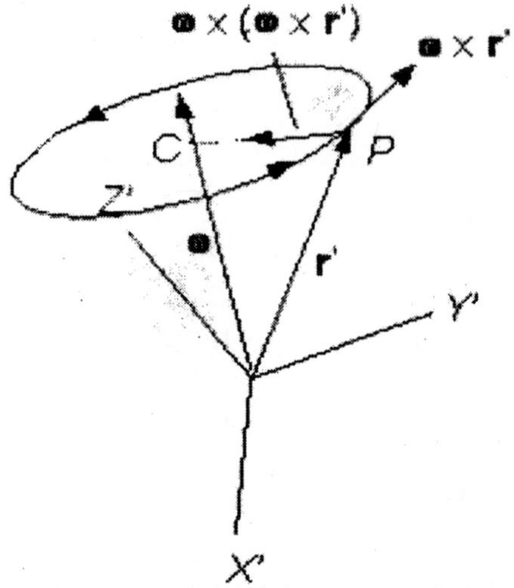

Figure 2

If the moving frame does not translate but rotates with a constant angular velocity and point *P* does not move within the moving frame, [4] can be simplified to

$$\mathbf{a} = \boldsymbol{\omega} \times (\boldsymbol{\omega} \times \mathbf{r}') \quad [5]$$

since

$$\mathbf{a}_0 = \dot{\boldsymbol{\omega}} = \mathbf{v}'_r = \mathbf{a}'_r = 0 \quad [6]$$

In order words, the centripetal acceleration is the basic requirement for a constant circular motion of a body around an axis of rotation. According to Newton's 2nd Law of Motion the force acting on a particle is equal to the its mass times acceleration. Therefore, from [6]:

$$\mathbf{F} = m\boldsymbol{\omega} \times (\boldsymbol{\omega} \times \mathbf{r}') \quad [7]$$

This force is the centripetal force which causes a constant circular motion of a body. Note that this force acts in the direction of the center of rotation, point *C* shown in Figure 2.

If the angular velocity of the rotating reference frame is not constant, [4] reduces to

$$\mathbf{a} = \dot{\boldsymbol{\omega}} \times \mathbf{r}' + \boldsymbol{\omega} \times (\boldsymbol{\omega} \times \mathbf{r}') \quad [8]$$

since

$$\mathbf{a}_o = \mathbf{v}'_r = \mathbf{a}'_r = 0 \quad [9]$$

In the case of planar rotation where the direction of the angular velocity does not change, the 1st term of [8] can be labeled as the **tangential acceleration** since it is in the direction of ω x **r'** shown in Figure 2. (The angular velocity vector and the angular acceleration vector show the same direction in this case.) The 2nd term then becomes the radial acceleration

Acceleration of a Rigid Body

In a rigid body shown in Figure 1, the position of point *P* relative to the moving reference frame fixed to the body remains constant, thus,

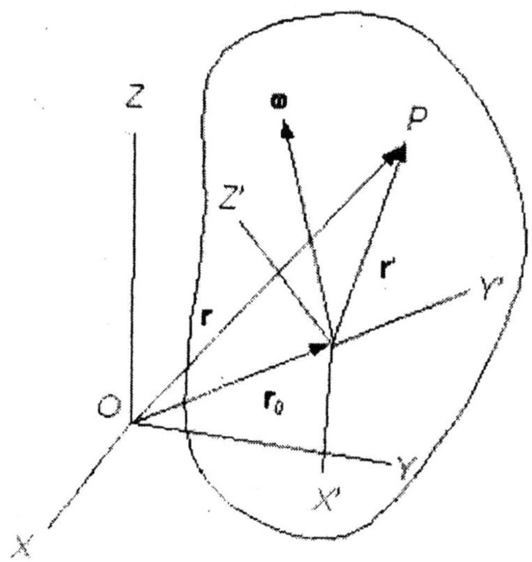

Figure 1

$$\mathbf{j}_P \times \mathbf{J}_P + \mathbf{m}_P \times \mathbf{M}_P = \dot{\mathbf{H}} - \mathbf{j}_D \times \mathbf{J}_D - \mathbf{m}_D \times \mathbf{M}_D - \mathbf{e} \times \mathbf{F}_E - \mathbf{T}_E \quad [4]$$

Since [3] and [4] together contain 3 groups of unknowns, **M**, **J**, and **m**, they provide an underdetermined system: number of the unknowns exceed that of the equations. In order to solve this system, one should either reduce the number of unknowns or add an equation to the system. Let's take the former strategy. Let

$$\mathbf{F} \equiv \mathbf{J} + \mathbf{M} \quad [5]$$

In other words, **F** is the sum of both the muscle force and the joint reaction force. Substitution of [5] into [3] and [4] yields

$$\mathbf{F}_P = \dot{\mathbf{p}} - \mathbf{F}_D - \mathbf{W} - \mathbf{F}_E \quad [6]$$

$$\mathbf{j}_P \times \mathbf{J}_P + \mathbf{j}_P \times \mathbf{M}_P - \mathbf{j}_P \times \mathbf{M}_P + \mathbf{m}_P \times \mathbf{M}_P$$
$$= \dot{\mathbf{H}} - \mathbf{j}_D \times \mathbf{J}_D - \mathbf{j}_D \times \mathbf{M}_D + \mathbf{j}_D \times \mathbf{M}_D - \mathbf{m}_D \times \mathbf{M}_D - \mathbf{e} \times \mathbf{F}_E - \mathbf{T}_E$$
$$\mathbf{j}_P \times \mathbf{F}_P + (\mathbf{m}_P - \mathbf{j}_P) \times \mathbf{M}_P = \dot{\mathbf{H}} - \mathbf{j}_D \times \mathbf{F}_D - (\mathbf{m}_D - \mathbf{j}_D) \times \mathbf{M}_D - \mathbf{e} \times \mathbf{F}_E - \mathbf{T}_E \quad [7]$$

Now, let

$$\mathbf{T} \equiv (\mathbf{m} - \mathbf{j}) \times \mathbf{M} \quad [8]$$

Using [8], one can reduce [7] to

$$\mathbf{j}_P \times \mathbf{F}_P + \mathbf{T}_P = \dot{\mathbf{H}} - \mathbf{j}_D \times \mathbf{F}_D - \mathbf{T}_D - \mathbf{e} \times \mathbf{F}_E - \mathbf{T}_E \quad [9]$$

[6] and [9] now have two groups of unknowns, **F** and **T**. Assuming that $\mathbf{F}_D$ and $\mathbf{T}_D$ are somehow known, one can solve the system for $\mathbf{F}_P$ and $\mathbf{T}_P$.

Joint Torque and Net Joint Force

Even though **F** and **T** in [6] and [9] were invented for computational convenience, these quantities may have some practical meaning.

Firstly, **T** is a sort of torque since it is in the form of (position vector) x (force). Since vector **m** - **j** is the relative position of the application point of **M** to the joint center, as shown on Figure 2, **T** becomes the torque produced by the muscle force about the joint center (**joint torque**). This quantity is meaningful since it gives the amount of torque produced by the muscle about the joint. On the other hand, **F** (**net joint force**) is simply the sum of **J** and **M** and it does not provide any specific information in terms of muscle activation or the stress on the bones involved in the articulation. Therefore, one must not give any major meaning to the net joint force (**F**) while interpreting data.

Figure 3 shows two equivalent systems with the new system represented by the joint torque and the net joint force. **M**, **J** and **m** are simply replaced by **F** and **T**. Again, circling arrows instead of straight arrows are used here as the torque vectors for better visual effect.

Solutions

Now, let's get back to [6] and [9]. In order to solve this system for $\mathbf{F}_P$ and $\mathbf{T}_P$, one must know $\mathbf{F}_D$ and $\mathbf{T}_D$. There are two possible cases:

There is no distal segment linked the current segment so that $\mathbf{F}_D = 0$ and $\mathbf{T}_D = 0$.

$\mathbf{F}_D$ and $\mathbf{T}_D$ are somehow known.

The foot segment is a good example of the first case. There is no segment linked to the foot distally as shown in Figure 4. [6] and [9] therefore reduce to

$$\mathbf{F}_{AK/FT} = \dot{\mathbf{P}}_{FT} - \mathbf{W}_{FT} - \mathbf{F}_{GRF} \quad [10]$$

$$\mathbf{T}_{AK/FT} = \dot{\mathbf{H}}_{FT} - \mathbf{e}_{GRF} \times \mathbf{F}_{GRF} - \mathbf{T}_{GRF} - \mathbf{j}_{AK/FT} \times \mathbf{F}_{AK/FT} \quad [11]$$

where $\mathbf{F}_{AK/FT}$ = the net joint force acting on the foot at the ankle, $\mathbf{T}_{AK/FT}$ = the joint torque produced by the muscles attached to the foot around the ankle, and $\mathbf{j}_{AK/FT}$ = the relative position vector of the ankle to the foot CM. *GRF* stands for the ground reaction force.

Now, let's move to the shank (Figure 5). In the shank, one can not ignore **F** and **T** at the distal end and this falls into the second case listed above. Assuming all muscles included in this model are uni-articular, one can come up with

$$\mathbf{F}_{AK/SH} = -\mathbf{F}_{AK/FT} \quad [12]$$

$$\mathbf{T}_{AK/SH} = -\mathbf{T}_{AK/FT} \quad [13]$$

Both [12] and [13] are obtained from the **Newton's 3rd Law of Motion: Law of Reaction**. "For every action there is an equal and opposite reaction."

As shown in Figure 6, muscle forces $\mathbf{M}_{AK/SH}$ and $\mathbf{M}_{AK/FT}$ have an action-reaction relationship since all muscles are uni-articular. They have the same moment arm about the ankle joint, thus torques $\mathbf{T}_{AK/SH}$ and $\mathbf{T}_{AK/FT}$ also have an action-reaction relationship.

Based on [12] and [13], one can reduce [6] and [9] to

$$\begin{aligned}\mathbf{F}_{KN/SH} &= \dot{\mathbf{p}}_{SH} - \mathbf{F}_{AK/SH} - \mathbf{W}_{SH} \\ &= \dot{\mathbf{p}}_{SH} + \mathbf{F}_{AK/FT} - \mathbf{W}_{SH} \quad [14]\end{aligned}$$

$$\begin{aligned}\mathbf{T}_{KN/SH} &= \dot{\mathbf{H}}_{SH} - \mathbf{j}_{AK/SH} \times \mathbf{F}_{AK/SH} - \mathbf{T}_{AK/SH} - \mathbf{j}_{KN/SH} \times \mathbf{F}_{KN/SH} \\ &= \dot{\mathbf{H}}_{SH} + \mathbf{j}_{AK/SH} \times \mathbf{F}_{AK/FT} + \mathbf{T}_{AK/FT} - \mathbf{j}_{KN/SH} \times \mathbf{F}_{KN/SH} \quad [15]\end{aligned}$$

where $\mathbf{F}_{KN/SH}$ = the net joint force acting on the shank at the knee, $\mathbf{T}_{KN/SH}$ = the joint torque produced by the muscles attached to the shank around the knee, $\mathbf{j}_{KN/SH}$ = the relative position vector of the knee to the shank CM, and $\mathbf{j}_{AK/SH}$ = the relative position vector of the ankle to the shank CM. Here, of course, it was assumed that there is no additional external force acting on the shank from the environment.

Similarly, the net joint force and the joint torque of the hip-thigh can be written as

$$\mathbf{F}_{HP/TH} = \dot{\mathbf{p}}_{TH} - \mathbf{F}_{KN/TH} - \mathbf{W}_{TH}$$
$$= \dot{\mathbf{p}}_{TH} + \mathbf{F}_{KN/SH} - \mathbf{W}_{TH} \quad [16]$$

$$\mathbf{T}_{HP/TH} = \dot{\mathbf{H}}_{TH} - \mathbf{j}_{KN/Th} \times \mathbf{F}_{KN/TH} - \mathbf{T}_{KN/TH} - \mathbf{j}_{HP/TH} \times \mathbf{F}_{HP/TH}$$
$$= \dot{\mathbf{H}}_{TH} + \mathbf{j}_{KN/TH} \times \mathbf{F}_{KN/SH} + \mathbf{T}_{KN/SH} - \mathbf{j}_{HP/TH} \times \mathbf{F}_{HP/TH}$$

[17]

Similar approach can be used in computing the joint torques of the arm joints, starting from the hand. For a complex whole body motion one must compute the joint torques using the sequence shown in Figure 7.

Rate of Change in Linear and Angular Momentum

The rates of change in momentum and angular momentum used in the equations can be computed based on the kinematic data obtained from motion analysis. The rate of change in linear momentum in [6] is

$$\dot{\mathbf{p}} = \frac{d(m\mathbf{v})}{dt} = m\mathbf{a} \quad [18]$$

where m = the mass of the segment, **a** = the acceleration of the segment CM. m can be obtained through the BSP estimation while **a** can be computed from the position of the segment CM.

The rate of change in angular momentum of the segment is the net torque acting on the segment:

$$\dot{\mathbf{H}} = \frac{d\mathbf{H}}{dt}$$

$$= \left(\frac{d\mathbf{H}}{dt}\right)_{rot} + \boldsymbol{\omega} \times \mathbf{H} = \begin{bmatrix} I_{xx}\dot{\omega}_x \\ I_{yy}\dot{\omega}_y \\ I_{zz}\dot{\omega}_z \end{bmatrix} + \begin{bmatrix} 0 & -\omega_z & \omega_y \\ \omega_z & 0 & -\omega_x \\ -\omega_y & \omega_x & 0 \end{bmatrix} \begin{bmatrix} I_{xx}\omega_x \\ I_{yy}\omega_y \\ I_{zz}\omega_z \end{bmatrix}$$

[19]

where $\boldsymbol{\omega}$ = the angular velocity of the segment, $()_{rot}$ = a vector observed in the rotating reference frame (segmental reference frame). See the Rotating Reference Frame section for the details. The inertia tensor of the segment (**I**), the angular velocity ($\boldsymbol{\omega}$), and the angular momentum of the segment (**H**) are given as

$$\mathbf{I} = \begin{bmatrix} I_{xx} & 0 & 0 \\ 0 & I_{yy} & 0 \\ 0 & 0 & I_{zz} \end{bmatrix}$$ **[20]**

$$\boldsymbol{\omega} = \begin{bmatrix} \omega_x \\ \omega_y \\ \omega_z \end{bmatrix}$$ **[21]**

$$\mathbf{H} = \mathbf{I}\boldsymbol{\omega} = \begin{bmatrix} I_{xx}\omega_x \\ I_{yy}\omega_y \\ I_{zz}\omega_z \end{bmatrix}$$ **[22]**

x, *y* & *z* in the equations stand for the three axes of the segment reference frame in rotation. Inertia tensor **I** can be obtained from the BSP data while $\boldsymbol{\omega}$ can be found through motion analysis. See the Angular Velocity vs. Orientation Angles page for the details of how to compute $\boldsymbol{\omega}$ using the orientation angles.

As shown in [19], one can compute the net torque of the segment from the inertia tensor and the angular velocity. One must not forget to transform the net torque vector to the global frame after the computation if all other vectors are described in the global frame. Another simple way to compute the net torque is to obtain it directly from the global angular momentum data through time-derivation.

The angular orientation angles can also be used in the computation of the angular velocity of the object. By taking the time-derivatives of the orientation angles, one can obtain three independent angular velocities: $\dot{\phi}, \dot{\theta}, \& \dot{\psi}$. One thing important here is the directions of the three angular velocity vectors. The direction of the first rotation ($\dot{\phi}$) is about the *X* / *X'* axis shown in Figure 1 while the second rotation ($\dot{\theta}$) is about the *Y'* / *Y"* axis. The third rotation ($\dot{\psi}$) is about the *Z"* / *Z'"* axis. For vector addition, it is necessary to transform the angular velocity vectors to a common reference frame:

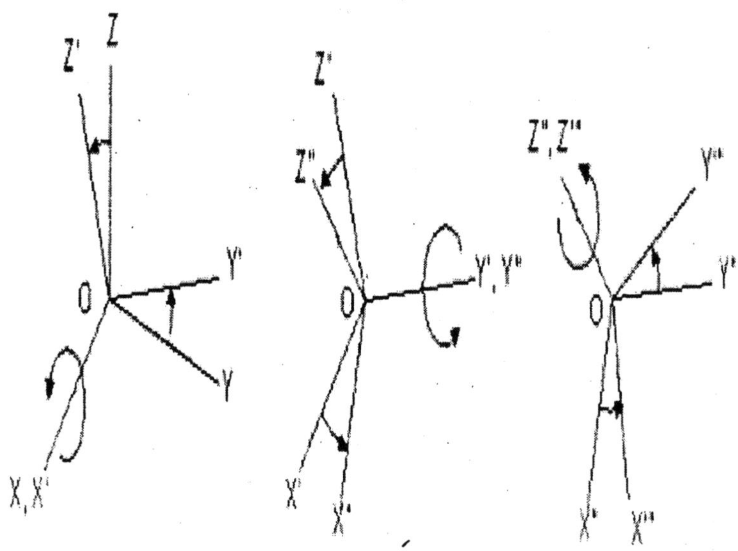

Figure 1

$$\boldsymbol{\omega}_{B/A}^{(B)} = \mathbf{R}_z(\psi)\cdot\mathbf{R}_y(\theta)\cdot\begin{bmatrix}\dot{\phi}\\0\\0\end{bmatrix} + \mathbf{R}_z(\psi)\cdot\begin{bmatrix}0\\\dot{\theta}\\0\end{bmatrix} + \begin{bmatrix}0\\0\\\dot{\psi}\end{bmatrix}$$

$$= \begin{bmatrix}c(\psi) & s(\psi) & 0\\-s(\psi) & c(\psi) & 0\\0 & 0 & 1\end{bmatrix}\begin{bmatrix}c(\theta) & 0 & -s(\theta)\\0 & 1 & 0\\s(\theta) & 0 & c(\theta)\end{bmatrix}\begin{bmatrix}\dot{\phi}\\0\\0\end{bmatrix} + \begin{bmatrix}c(\psi) & s(\psi) & 0\\-s(\psi) & c(\psi) & 0\\0 & 0 & 1\end{bmatrix}\begin{bmatrix}0\\\dot{\theta}\\0\end{bmatrix} + \begin{bmatrix}0\\0\\\dot{\psi}\end{bmatrix}$$

$$= \begin{bmatrix}c(\theta)c(\psi) & s(\psi) & 0\\-c(\theta)s(\psi) & c(\psi) & 0\\s(\theta) & 0 & 1\end{bmatrix}\begin{bmatrix}\dot{\phi}\\\dot{\theta}\\\dot{\psi}\end{bmatrix}$$

[1]

or

$$\boldsymbol{\omega}_{B/A}^{(A)} = \begin{bmatrix}\dot{\phi}\\0\\0\end{bmatrix} + \mathbf{R}_x(-\phi)\cdot\begin{bmatrix}0\\\dot{\theta}\\0\end{bmatrix} + \mathbf{R}_x(-\phi)\cdot\mathbf{R}_y(-\theta)\cdot\begin{bmatrix}0\\0\\\dot{\psi}\end{bmatrix}$$

$$= \begin{bmatrix}\dot{\phi}\\0\\0\end{bmatrix} + \begin{bmatrix}1 & 0 & 0\\0 & c(\phi) & -s(\phi)\\0 & s(\phi) & c(\phi)\end{bmatrix}\begin{bmatrix}0\\\dot{\theta}\\0\end{bmatrix} + \begin{bmatrix}1 & 0 & 0\\0 & c(\phi) & -s(\phi)\\0 & s(\phi) & c(\phi)\end{bmatrix}\begin{bmatrix}c(\theta) & 0 & s(\theta)\\0 & 1 & 0\\-s(\theta) & 0 & c(\theta)\end{bmatrix}\begin{bmatrix}0\\0\\\dot{\psi}\end{bmatrix}$$

$$= \begin{bmatrix}1 & 0 & s(\theta)\\0 & c(\phi) & -s(\phi)c(\theta)\\0 & s(\phi) & c(\phi)c(\theta)\end{bmatrix}\begin{bmatrix}\dot{\phi}\\\dot{\theta}\\\dot{\psi}\end{bmatrix}$$

[2]

where, $\omega_{B/A}$ = the angular velocity of frame *B* relative to frame *A*, and ϕ, θ, and ψ = the three orientation angles of frame *B* relative to frame *A*. [10] shows the angular velocity of frame *B* relative to *A* described in frame *B* while [11] shows the same vector described in frame *A*. Choose the right form of angular velocity depending on your needs. If the global angular velocity of frame *A* (ω_A) is available, the actual angular velocity of frame *B* is

$$\omega_B = T_{A/G}^{\,t} \cdot \omega_{B/A}^{(A)} + \omega_A$$

$$\omega_B = T_{B/G}^{\,t} \cdot \omega_{B/A}^{(B)} + \omega_A \quad [3]$$

Transformation Matrix

Electromagnetic motion sensors such as Flock of Bird® (Ascension Technology Corporation, Burlington, VT) generate positions and orientations of the sensors (birds) in real time. According to the manual (Ascension Technology Corporation, 1999), the rotation matrix the system produces is basically the ZYX type:

$$\mathbf{R} = \begin{bmatrix} 1 & 0 & 0 \\ 0 & c(\xi) & s(\xi) \\ 0 & -s(\xi) & c(\xi) \end{bmatrix} \begin{bmatrix} c(\psi) & 0 & -s(\psi) \\ 0 & 1 & 0 \\ s(\psi) & 0 & c(\psi) \end{bmatrix} \begin{bmatrix} c(\zeta) & s(\zeta) & 0 \\ -s(\zeta) & c(\zeta) & 0 \\ 0 & 0 & 1 \end{bmatrix}$$

$$= \begin{bmatrix} 1 & 0 & 0 \\ 0 & c(\xi) & s(\xi) \\ 0 & -s(\xi) & c(\xi) \end{bmatrix} \begin{bmatrix} c(\psi)c(\zeta) & c(\psi)s(\zeta) & -s(\psi) \\ -s(\zeta) & c(\zeta) & 0 \\ s(\psi)c(\zeta) & s(\psi)s(\zeta) & c(\psi) \end{bmatrix}$$

$$= \begin{bmatrix} c(\psi)c(\zeta) & c(\psi)s(\zeta) & -s(\psi) \\ -c(\xi)s(\zeta)+s(\xi)s(\psi)c(\zeta) & c(\xi)c(\zeta)+s(\xi)s(\psi)s(\zeta) & s(\xi)c(\psi) \\ s(\xi)s(\zeta)+c(\xi)s(\psi)c(\zeta) & -s(\xi)c(\zeta)+c(\xi)s(\psi)s(\zeta) & c(\xi)c(\psi) \end{bmatrix}$$

, **[1]**

where ξ, ψ, and ζ = the rotation angles about the *X*, *Y*, and *Z* axis, respectively. This rotation matrix can be applied to a 3-D image to make it follow the rotation of the sensor. In other words, this matrix the transformation matrix from the sensor reference frame to the transmitter reference frame:

$$\mathbf{T}_{T/S} = \begin{bmatrix} c(\psi)c(\zeta) & c(\psi)s(\zeta) & -s(\psi) \\ -c(\xi)s(\zeta)+s(\xi)s(\psi)c(\zeta) & c(\xi)c(\zeta)+s(\xi)s(\psi)s(\zeta) & s(\xi)c(\psi) \\ s(\xi)s(\zeta)+c(\xi)s(\psi)c(\zeta) & -s(\xi)c(\zeta)+c(\xi)s(\psi)s(\zeta) & c(\xi)c(\psi) \end{bmatrix}$$

[2]

where S = the current sensor, and T = the transmitter. The transformation matrix from the transmitter frame to the sensor frame can be described as

$$\mathbf{T}_{S/T} = \mathbf{T}_{T/S}{}^{t}$$

$$= \begin{bmatrix} c(\psi)c(\zeta) & -c(\xi)s(\zeta)+s(\xi)s(\psi)c(\zeta) & s(\xi)s(\zeta)+c(\xi)s(\psi)c(\zeta) \\ c(\psi)s(\zeta) & c(\xi)c(\zeta)+s(\xi)s(\psi)s(\zeta) & -s(\xi)c(\zeta)+c(\xi)s(\psi)s(\zeta) \\ -s(\psi) & s(\xi)c(\psi) & c(\xi)c(\psi) \end{bmatrix}$$

[3]

Comparison of [3] above and [3] in the Orientation Angles page reveals the the following relationship:

$$\phi = -\xi$$
$$\theta = -\psi$$
$$\psi = -\zeta \quad \textbf{[4]}$$

These relationships basically summarize the nature of the rotation angles produced by FOB: the relative orientation angles of the transmitter reference frame to the sensor reference frame. Thus, the transformation matrix from the transmitter reference frame to the sensor reference frame is the *XYZ*-type with the orientation angles being $-\xi$, $-\psi$, and $-\zeta$, respectively.

One problem is the direction of the axes of the transmitter reference frame. The transmitter of the MotionStar® uses a rather unusual axis setup (Fig. 1). Assuming the Y-axis of the transmitter reference frame is aligned with that of the desired global reference frame, the relationship between the transmitter reference frame and the global reference frame can be summarized as

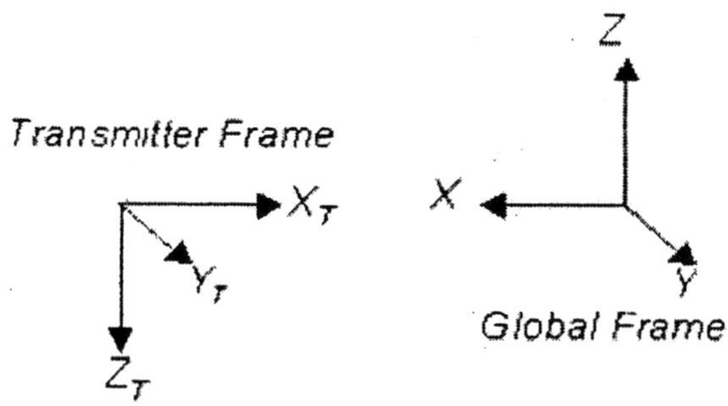

Fig. 1

$$\mathbf{T}_{G/T} = \begin{bmatrix} \cos\pi & 0 & -\sin\pi \\ 0 & 1 & 0 \\ \sin\pi & 0 & \cos\pi \end{bmatrix} = \begin{bmatrix} -1 & 0 & 0 \\ 0 & 1 & 0 \\ 0 & 0 & -1 \end{bmatrix}, \quad [5]$$

where T = the transmitter reference frame, and G = the global frame. Also from [5]:

$$\mathbf{T}_{T/G} = \mathbf{T}_{G/T}{}^{t} = \begin{bmatrix} -1 & 0 & 0 \\ 0 & 1 & 0 \\ 0 & 0 & -1 \end{bmatrix}. \quad [6]$$

The transformation matrix from the sensor reference frame to the global reference frame is then

$$\mathbf{T}_{G/S} = \mathbf{T}_{G/T} \cdot \mathbf{T}_{T/S} = \begin{bmatrix} -1 & 0 & 0 \\ 0 & 1 & 0 \\ 0 & 0 & -1 \end{bmatrix} \cdot \mathbf{T}_{T/S} \quad [7]$$

Likewise, the transformation from the global frame to the sensor reference frame is

$$\mathbf{T}_{S/G} = \mathbf{T}_{S/T} \cdot \mathbf{T}_{T/G}$$
$$= \mathbf{T}_{T/S}{}^{t} \cdot \begin{bmatrix} -1 & 0 & 0 \\ 0 & 1 & 0 \\ 0 & 0 & -1 \end{bmatrix} \qquad [8]$$

Transformation from one sensor reference frame (*A*) to another (*B*) can be written as

$$\mathbf{T}_{B/A} = \mathbf{T}_{B/G} \cdot \mathbf{T}_{G/A}$$
$$= \mathbf{T}_{G/B}{}^{t} \cdot \mathbf{T}_{G/A}$$
$$= \left[\begin{bmatrix} -1 & 0 & 0 \\ 0 & 1 & 0 \\ 0 & 0 & -1 \end{bmatrix} \cdot \mathbf{T}_{T/B} \right]^{t} \cdot \begin{bmatrix} -1 & 0 & 0 \\ 0 & 1 & 0 \\ 0 & 0 & -1 \end{bmatrix} \cdot \mathbf{T}_{T/A}$$
$$= \mathbf{T}_{T/B}{}^{t} \cdot \mathbf{T}_{T/A}$$
$$\mathbf{T}_{B/A} = \mathbf{T}_{B/T} \cdot \mathbf{T}_{T/A} = \mathbf{T}_{T/B}{}^{t} \cdot \mathbf{T}_{T/A} \qquad , [9]$$

where matrices $\mathbf{T}_{T/A}$ and $\mathbf{T}_{T/B}$ are the direct output of the system. Pay attention to the direction of the axes of the sensor reference frame.

Position of the Sensors

The positions of the sensors reported by the electromagnetic system are basically described in the transmitter reference frame. Thus, the global position of a sensor (*S*) can be described as:

$$\mathbf{r}_S = \begin{bmatrix} -1 & 0 & 0 \\ 0 & 1 & 0 \\ 0 & 0 & -1 \end{bmatrix} \cdot \mathbf{r}_S^{(T)} + \mathbf{r}_T \quad , \quad [10]$$

where $\mathbf{r}_S$ = the global position of the sensor, $\mathbf{r}_S^{(T)}$ = the relative position of the sensor to the transmitter described in the transmitter reference frame (the immediate output of the sensor system), and $\mathbf{r}_T$ = the global position of the transmitter.

Functional Method

The functional method is useful in locating the center of rotation of a ball-and-socket joint or the axis of rotation of a hinge joint. It computes the center/axis of rotation numerically rather than relying on a set of predetermined ratios or prediction equations.

The hip joint is a ball-and-socket joint and has 3 degrees of freedom. In an ideal situation, markers attached to the thigh will form spheres with the hip joint being the center if the pelvis is stationary. Thus, it is possible to numerically compute the center of the spheres based on the marker coordinates.

Four methods (algorithms) are included in this page: 2 closed-form least square algorithms by HU Gamage & Lasenby (2002), and Halvorsen et al. (1999), respectively, the Nelder-Mead downhill simplex method, and the Newton's method.

Fig. 1 shows the geometric relationship between the hip joint and the markers attached to the thigh. Each marker on the thigh will form a sphere with the hip joint being its center. Vector $\mathbf{r}_c$ in Fig. 1 is the position of the hip joint center while vector $\mathbf{r}_{ji}$ is the position of marker *j* at frame *i*.

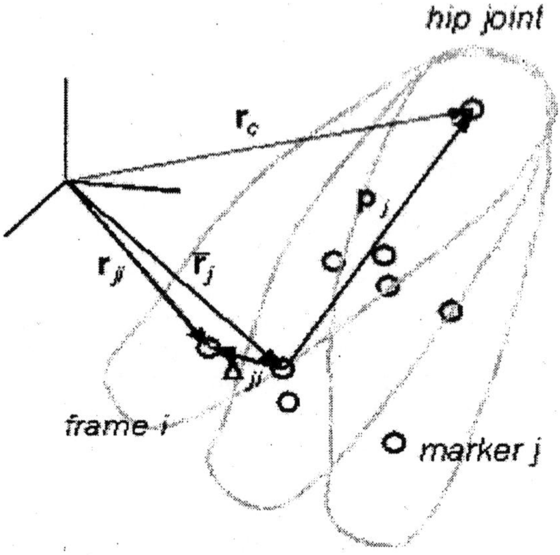

[Fig. 1]

The error function ε_{ji} can be defined as

$$\varepsilon_{ji} = (\mathbf{r}_{ji} - \mathbf{r}_c)\cdot(\mathbf{r}_{ji} - \mathbf{r}_c) - R_j^2, \quad \textbf{[1]}$$

where R_j = radius of the sphere formed by marker *j*. Thus, the cost function for the least square approximation of the hip joint center becomes

$$U = \sum_{j=1}^{m}\sum_{i=1}^{n} \varepsilon_{ji}^2 = \sum_{j=1}^{m}\sum_{i=1}^{n}\left[(\mathbf{r}_{ji} - \mathbf{r}_c)\cdot(\mathbf{r}_{ji} - \mathbf{r}_c) - R_j^2\right]^2 \quad \textbf{[2]}$$

The cost function U in [1] must be minimized to obtain the position of the center of the spheres (hip joint).

Now, let's define the mean position of marker *j* shown in Fig. 1 as:

$$\overline{\mathbf{r}}_j = \frac{1}{n}\sum_{i=1}^{n}\mathbf{r}_{ji} \quad \textbf{[3]}$$

The relative position of the marker to the mean position at frame *i* can be expressed in terms of the mean position:

$$\mathbf{\Delta}_{ji} = \mathbf{r}_{ji} - \overline{\mathbf{r}}_j, \quad [4]$$

where

$$\sum_{j=1}^{n} \mathbf{\Delta}_{ji} = 0 \quad [5]$$

Vector $\mathbf{p}_j$ shown in Fig. 1 is the relative position of the joint center to the mean position of marker *j*:

$$\mathbf{p}_j = \mathbf{r}_c - \overline{\mathbf{r}}_j. \quad [6]$$

Therefore:

$$\mathbf{r}_c = \mathbf{p}_j + \overline{\mathbf{r}}_j$$

$$\mathbf{r}_{ji} - \mathbf{r}_c = \left(\mathbf{\Delta}_i + \overline{\mathbf{r}}_j\right) - \left(\overline{\mathbf{r}}_j + \mathbf{p}_j\right) = \mathbf{\Delta}_{ji} - \mathbf{p}_j \quad [7]$$

The cost function shown in [1] can be then rewritten as

$$U = \sum_{j=1}^{m} \sum_{i=1}^{n} \left[\left(\mathbf{\Delta}_{ji} - \mathbf{p}_j\right) \cdot \left(\mathbf{\Delta}_{ji} - \mathbf{p}_j\right) - R_j^2\right]^2 \quad [8]$$

Minimization of the cost function *U* yields

$$\frac{\partial U}{\partial R_j} = 0 \quad [9]$$

and

$$\frac{\partial U}{\partial \mathbf{p}_j} = 0$$ **[10]**

From [9]:

$$\frac{\partial U}{\partial R_j} = 0 = -4R_j \sum_{i=1}^{n} \left[\left(\mathbf{\Delta}_{ji} - \mathbf{p}_j \right) \cdot \left(\mathbf{\Delta}_{ji} - \mathbf{p}_j \right) - R_j^2 \right]$$

$$0 = \sum_{i=1}^{n} \left[\left(\mathbf{\Delta}_{ji} - \mathbf{p}_j \right) \cdot \left(\mathbf{\Delta}_{ji} - \mathbf{p}_j \right) - R_j^2 \right]$$ **[11]**

where $R_j \neq 0$

From [10]:

$$\frac{\partial U}{\partial \mathbf{p}_j} = 0 = -4 \sum_{i=1}^{n} \left[\left(\mathbf{\Delta}_{ji} - \mathbf{p}_j \right) \cdot \left(\mathbf{\Delta}_{ji} - \mathbf{p}_j \right) - R_j^2 \right] \left(\mathbf{\Delta}_{ji} - \mathbf{p}_j \right)$$

$$\begin{aligned}
0 &= \sum_{i=1}^{n} \left[\left(\mathbf{\Delta}_{ji} - \mathbf{p}_j \right) \cdot \left(\mathbf{\Delta}_{ji} - \mathbf{p}_j \right) - R_j^2 \right] \left(\mathbf{\Delta}_{ji} - \mathbf{p}_j \right) \\
&= \sum_{i=1}^{n} \left[\left(\mathbf{\Delta}_{ji} - \mathbf{p}_j \right) \cdot \left(\mathbf{\Delta}_{ji} - \mathbf{p}_j \right) \right] \mathbf{\Delta}_{ji} - R_j^2 \sum_{i=1}^{n} \mathbf{\Delta}_{ji} - \mathbf{p}_j \sum_{i=1}^{n} \left[\left(\mathbf{\Delta}_{ji} - \mathbf{p}_j \right) \cdot \left(\mathbf{\Delta}_{ji} - \mathbf{p}_j \right) - R_j^2 \right] \\
&= \sum_{i=1}^{n} \left[\left(\mathbf{\Delta}_{ji} - \mathbf{p}_j \right) \cdot \left(\mathbf{\Delta}_{ji} - \mathbf{p}_j \right) \right] \mathbf{\Delta}_{ji} \\
&= \sum_{i=1}^{n} \left[\mathbf{\Delta}_{ji} \cdot \mathbf{\Delta}_{ji} - 2\mathbf{\Delta}_{ji} \cdot \mathbf{p}_j + \mathbf{p}_j \cdot \mathbf{p}_j \right] \mathbf{\Delta}_{ji} \\
&= \sum_{i=1}^{n} \left(\mathbf{\Delta}_{ji} \cdot \mathbf{\Delta}_{ji} \right) \mathbf{\Delta}_{ji} - 2 \sum_{i=1}^{n} \left(\mathbf{\Delta}_{ji} \cdot \mathbf{p}_j \right) \mathbf{\Delta}_{ji} + \mathbf{p}_j \cdot \mathbf{p}_j \sum_{i=1}^{n} \mathbf{\Delta}_{ji} \\
&= \sum_{i=1}^{n} \left(\mathbf{\Delta}_{ji} \cdot \mathbf{\Delta}_{ji} \right) \mathbf{\Delta}_{ji} - 2 \sum_{i=1}^{n} \mathbf{\Delta}_{ji} \left(\mathbf{\Delta}_{ji} \cdot \mathbf{p}_j \right)
\end{aligned}$$

12]

Note that [5] and [11] were used in deriving [12]. From [12]:

$$2\sum_{j=1}^{n}\boldsymbol{\Delta}_{ji}\left(\boldsymbol{\Delta}_{ji}\cdot\mathbf{p}_j\right)=\sum_{j=1}^{n}\boldsymbol{\Delta}_{ji}\left(\boldsymbol{\Delta}_{ji}\cdot\boldsymbol{\Delta}_{ji}\right) \qquad [13]$$

Rewrite [13] in the matrix form and divide both sides by *n*:

$$2\frac{1}{n}\sum_{i=1}^{n}\{\boldsymbol{\Delta}_{ji}\}\{\boldsymbol{\Delta}_{ji}\}^t\{\mathbf{p}_j\}=\frac{1}{n}\sum_{i=1}^{n}\{\boldsymbol{\Delta}_{ji}\}\{\boldsymbol{\Delta}_{ji}\}^t\{\boldsymbol{\Delta}_{ji}\} \qquad [14]$$

where { } = column matrix of the vector. [14] basically has the following form:

$$\mathbf{A}_j\{\mathbf{p}_j\}=\mathbf{B}_j, \qquad [15]$$

where

$$\begin{aligned}\mathbf{A}_j&=\frac{2}{n}\sum_{i=1}^{n}\{\boldsymbol{\Delta}_{ji}\}\{\boldsymbol{\Delta}_{ji}\}^t=\frac{2}{n}\sum_{i=1}^{n}\{\mathbf{r}_{ji}-\bar{\mathbf{r}}_j\}\{\mathbf{r}_{ji}-\bar{\mathbf{r}}_j\}^t\\&=\frac{2}{n}\sum_{i=1}^{n}\left[\{\mathbf{r}_{ji}\}\{\mathbf{r}_{ji}\}^t-2\{\mathbf{r}_{ji}\}\{\bar{\mathbf{r}}_j\}^t+\{\bar{\mathbf{r}}_j\}\{\bar{\mathbf{r}}_j\}^t\right]\\&=\frac{2}{n}\left[\sum_{i=1}^{n}\{\mathbf{r}_{ji}\}\{\mathbf{r}_{ji}\}^t-2\sum_{i=1}^{n}\{\mathbf{r}_{ji}\}\{\bar{\mathbf{r}}_j\}^t+n\{\bar{\mathbf{r}}_j\}\{\bar{\mathbf{r}}_j\}^t\right]\\&=2\left[\frac{1}{n}\sum_{i=1}^{n}\{\mathbf{r}_{ji}\}\{\mathbf{r}_{ji}\}^t-\{\bar{\mathbf{r}}_j\}\{\bar{\mathbf{r}}_j\}^t\right]\end{aligned} \qquad [16]$$

and

$$\mathbf{B}_j = \frac{1}{n}\sum_{i=1}^{n}\{\Delta_{ji}\}\{\Delta_{ji}\}^t\{\Delta_{ji}\} = \frac{1}{n}\sum_{i=1}^{n}\{\mathbf{r}_{ji}-\bar{\mathbf{r}}_j\}\{\mathbf{r}_{ji}-\bar{\mathbf{r}}_j\}^t\{\mathbf{r}_{ji}-\bar{\mathbf{r}}_j\}$$

$$= \frac{1}{n}\sum_{i=1}^{n}\{\mathbf{r}_{ji}-\bar{\mathbf{r}}_j\}\left[\{\mathbf{r}_{ji}\}^t\{\mathbf{r}_{ji}\} - 2\{\mathbf{r}_{ji}\}^t\{\bar{\mathbf{r}}_j\} + \{\bar{\mathbf{r}}_j\}^t\{\bar{\mathbf{r}}_j\}\right]$$

$$= \frac{1}{n}\sum_{i=1}^{n}\left[\{\mathbf{r}_{ji}\}\{\mathbf{r}_{ji}\}^t\{\mathbf{r}_{ji}\} - 2\{\mathbf{r}_{ji}\}\{\mathbf{r}_{ji}\}^t\{\bar{\mathbf{r}}_j\} + \{\mathbf{r}_{ji}\}\{\bar{\mathbf{r}}_j\}^t\{\bar{\mathbf{r}}_j\}\right] - \{\bar{\mathbf{r}}_j\}\sum_{i=1}^{n}\left[\{\mathbf{r}_{ji}\}^t\{\mathbf{r}_{ji}\} - 2\{\mathbf{r}_{ji}\}^t\{\bar{\mathbf{r}}_j\} + \{\bar{\mathbf{r}}_j\}^t\{\bar{\mathbf{r}}_j\}\right]$$

$$= \frac{1}{n}\sum_{i=1}^{n}\{\mathbf{r}_{ji}\}\{\mathbf{r}_{ji}\}^t\{\mathbf{r}_{ji}\} - 2\left[\frac{1}{n}\sum_{i=1}^{n}\{\mathbf{r}_{ji}\}\{\mathbf{r}_{ji}\}^t\right]\{\bar{\mathbf{r}}_j\} + \left[\frac{1}{n}\sum_{i=1}^{n}\{\mathbf{r}_{ji}\}\right]\{\bar{\mathbf{r}}_j\}^t\{\bar{\mathbf{r}}_j\} - \{\bar{\mathbf{r}}_j\}\left[\frac{1}{n}\sum_{i=1}^{n}\{\mathbf{r}_{ji}\}^t\{\mathbf{r}_{ji}\}\right] + \{\bar{\mathbf{r}}_j\}\{\bar{\mathbf{r}}_j\}^t\{\bar{\mathbf{r}}_j\}$$

$$= \left[\frac{1}{n}\sum_{i=1}^{n}\{\mathbf{r}_{ji}\}\{\mathbf{r}_{ji}\}^t\{\mathbf{r}_{ji}\}\right] - \{\bar{\mathbf{r}}_j\}\left[\frac{1}{n}\sum_{i=1}^{n}\{\mathbf{r}_{ji}\}^t\{\mathbf{r}_{ji}\}\right] - 2\left[\frac{1}{n}\sum_{i=1}^{n}\{\mathbf{r}_{ji}\}\{\mathbf{r}_{ji}\}^t\right]\{\bar{\mathbf{r}}_j\} + 2\{\bar{\mathbf{r}}_j\}\{\bar{\mathbf{r}}_j\}^t\{\bar{\mathbf{r}}_j\}$$

[17]

$\mathbf{A}_j$ = (3 x 3) while $\mathbf{B}_j$ = (3 x 1). From [15], [16], and [17]:

$$2\left[\frac{1}{n}\sum_{i=1}^{n}\{\mathbf{r}_{ji}\}\{\mathbf{r}_{ji}\}^{t}-\{\bar{\mathbf{r}}_{j}\}\{\bar{\mathbf{r}}_{j}\}^{t}\right]\{\mathbf{r}_{c}\}=\left[\frac{1}{n}\sum_{i=1}^{n}\{\mathbf{r}_{ji}\}\{\mathbf{r}_{ji}\}^{t}\{\mathbf{r}_{ji}\}\right]-\{\bar{\mathbf{r}}_{j}\}\left[\frac{1}{n}\sum_{i=1}^{n}\{\mathbf{r}_{ji}\}^{t}\{\mathbf{r}_{ji}\}\right]$$
$$-2\left[\frac{1}{n}\sum_{i=1}^{n}\{\mathbf{r}_{ji}\}\{\mathbf{r}_{ji}\}^{t}\right]\{\bar{\mathbf{r}}_{j}\}+2\{\bar{\mathbf{r}}_{j}\}\{\bar{\mathbf{r}}_{j}\}^{t}\{\bar{\mathbf{r}}_{j}\}$$
$$+2\left[\frac{1}{n}\sum_{i=1}^{n}\{\mathbf{r}_{ji}\}\{\mathbf{r}_{ji}\}^{t}\right]\{\bar{\mathbf{r}}_{j}\}-2\{\bar{\mathbf{r}}_{j}\}\{\bar{\mathbf{r}}_{j}\}^{t}\{\bar{\mathbf{r}}_{j}\}$$
$$=\left[\frac{1}{n}\sum_{i=1}^{n}\{\mathbf{r}_{ji}\}\{\mathbf{r}_{ji}\}^{t}\{\mathbf{r}_{ji}\}\right]-\{\bar{\mathbf{r}}_{j}\}\left[\frac{1}{n}\sum_{i=1}^{n}\{\mathbf{r}_{ji}\}^{t}\{\mathbf{r}_{ji}\}\right]$$

[18]

[18] is basically in the form of

$$\mathbf{C}_j\{\mathbf{r}_c\}=\mathbf{D}_j\,, \quad \textbf{[19]}$$

where

$$\mathbf{C}_j=2\left[\frac{1}{n}\sum_{i=1}^{n}\{\mathbf{r}_{ji}\}\{\mathbf{r}_{ji}\}^{t}-\{\bar{\mathbf{r}}_{j}\}\{\bar{\mathbf{r}}_{j}\}^{t}\right]$$
$$\mathbf{D}_j=\left[\frac{1}{n}\sum_{i=1}^{n}\{\mathbf{r}_{ji}\}\{\mathbf{r}_{ji}\}^{t}\{\mathbf{r}_{ji}\}\right]-\{\bar{\mathbf{r}}_{j}\}\left[\frac{1}{n}\sum_{i=1}^{n}\{\mathbf{r}_{ji}\}^{t}\{\mathbf{r}_{ji}\}\right] \quad \textbf{[20]}$$

Expand [19] and [20] to all markers:

$$\mathbf{C}\{\mathbf{r}_c\} = \mathbf{D}$$

$$\mathbf{C} = \sum_{j=1}^{m} \mathbf{C}_j = 2\sum_{j=1}^{m}\left[\frac{1}{n}\sum_{i=1}^{n}\{\mathbf{r}_{ji}\}\{\mathbf{r}_{ji}\}^t - \{\bar{\mathbf{r}}_j\}\{\bar{\mathbf{r}}_j\}^t\right]$$

$$\mathbf{D} = \sum_{j=1}^{m} \mathbf{D}_j = \sum_{j=1}^{m}\left[\frac{1}{n}\sum_{i=1}^{n}\{\mathbf{r}_{ji}\}\{\mathbf{r}_{ji}\}^t\{\mathbf{r}_{ji}\}\right] - \sum_{j=1}^{m}\{\bar{\mathbf{r}}_j\}\left[\frac{1}{n}\sum_{i=1}^{n}\{\mathbf{r}_{ji}\}^t\{\mathbf{r}_{ji}\}\right]$$

, **[21]**

where **C** = (3 x 3) while **D** = (3 x 1). [19] is a linear system of equations of the position of the hip joint.

From [21]:

$$\{\mathbf{r}_c\} = \mathbf{C}^{-1}\,\mathbf{D}$$ **[22]**

This method was introduced by H. U. Gamage and Lasenby (2002). The advantage of this method is that it can handle multiple markers at once. The basic assumption is that the spheres formed by the markers have a common center (hip joint).

Nelder-Mead Downhill Simplex Method

Another algorithm that can be used in finding the hip joint center is the so-called **downhill simplex method** following Nelder and Mead. This method performs multidimensional minimization of the given function. In other words, it finds the minimum of the given cost function and the corresponding position of the hip joint center. Since this method does not involve derivatives, the cost function can be written as either

$$U = \sum_{j=1}^{m}\sum_{i=1}^{n}\left(\left|\mathbf{r}_{ji} - \mathbf{r}_c\right| - \frac{1}{n}\sum_{k=1}^{n}\left|\mathbf{r}_{jk} - \mathbf{r}_c\right|\right)^2$$ **[23]**

or

$$U=\sum_{j=1}^{m}\sum_{i=1}^{n}\left((\mathbf{r}_{ji}-\mathbf{r}_c)\cdot(\mathbf{r}_{ji}-\mathbf{r}_c)-\frac{1}{n}\sum_{k=1}^{n}(\mathbf{r}_{jk}-\mathbf{r}_c)\cdot(\mathbf{r}_{jk}-\mathbf{r}_c)\right)^2 \quad [24]$$

Although [24] looks more complex than [23], it requires less computations since the magnitude of a vector is typically computed from its square. $\mathbf{r}_c$ that minimizes U is the position of the hip.

The uniqueness of this method is in the method of systematic perturbation of $\mathbf{r}_c$ through iterations in multi dimensions to obtain the minimum of function U. It uses the so-called simplex for this and **tetrahedron** defined by 4 vertices (points) is the simplex in three-dimension. In other words, four position vectors instead of one will be used in obtaining the position of the hip joint center. If $\mathbf{p}_o$, the initial guess of $\mathbf{r}_c$, is available, the four vertices of the starting simplex can be given as

$$\begin{aligned}\mathbf{v}_o &= \mathbf{p}_o\\ \mathbf{v}_1 &= \mathbf{p}_o+\lambda\mathbf{i}\\ \mathbf{v}_2 &= \mathbf{p}_o+\lambda\mathbf{j}\\ \mathbf{v}_3 &= \mathbf{p}_o+\lambda\mathbf{k},\end{aligned} \quad [25]$$

where λ = constant, and **i**, **j**, & **k** = unit vectors of the axes. For example, the overall mean position of the markers can be used as the initial guess.

Each iteration consists of the following steps:

1. Identification of the vertices that provide the largest, second largest, and smallest function value: high, next high, and low point, respectively.
2. Convergence check. If it is sufficiently converged, read the low point coordinates as the hip joint center and stop the iterations.

3. Total number of iterations. See if it exceeded the maximum allowed. If yes, stop the iterations.
4. Determination of the type of simplex manipulation (Fig.2). Fig. 2a shows the simplex at the start of the current iteration.

[Fig. 2]

There are 6 different types of simplex manipulations possible:

a. Reflection: moving the high point through the opposite face to a lower point (Fig. 2b) or

$$\mathbf{v}_r = \left(\bar{\mathbf{v}} - \mathbf{v}_j\right) + \bar{\mathbf{v}}$$
$$\bar{\mathbf{v}} = \frac{1}{3}\sum_{i=0}^{3}\left(1-\delta_{ij}\right)\mathbf{v}_i \quad , \quad \textbf{[26]}$$

where $\mathbf{v}_r$ = reflected vertex position, j = the high point, δ_{ij} = Kronecker delta, and $\mathbf{v}$ = vertex position.

b. Reflection & expansion (Fig. 2c): extrapolation of the reflected point by a factor of 2, or

$$\mathbf{v}_{re} = 2\left(\bar{\mathbf{v}} - \mathbf{v}_j\right) + \bar{\mathbf{v}} \quad , \quad \textbf{[27]}$$

where $\mathbf{v}_{re}$ = reflected and expanded vertex position.

c. Contraction (Fig. 2d): one-dimensional contraction of the high point toward the opposite face, or

$$\mathbf{v}_c = \frac{1}{2}\left(\mathbf{v}_j - \bar{\mathbf{v}}\right) + \bar{\mathbf{v}} \quad , \quad \textbf{[28]}$$

where $\mathbf{v}_c$ = contracted vertex position.

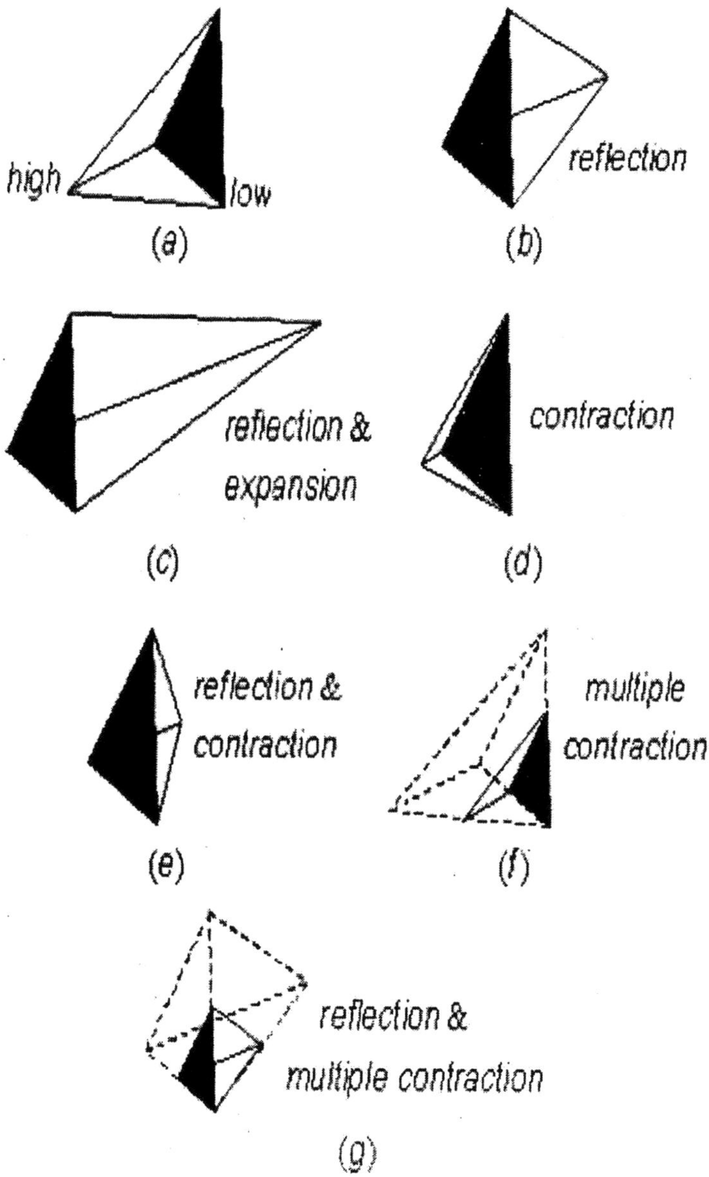
high
low
(a)
reflection
(b)
reflection &
expansion
(c)
contraction
(d)
reflection &
contraction
(e)
multiple
contraction
(f)
reflection &
multiple contraction
(g)

d. Reflection & contraction (Fig. 2e): one-dimensional contraction of the reflected point, or

$$\mathbf{v}_{rc} = \frac{1}{2}\left(\bar{\mathbf{v}} - \mathbf{v}_j\right) + \bar{\mathbf{v}} \quad , \quad [29]$$

where $\mathbf{v}_{rc}$ = reflected and contracted vertex position.

e. Multiple contraction (Fig. 2f): multi-dimensional contraction of the vertices toward the low point, or

$$\mathbf{v}_{mci} = \left(1 - \delta_{ik}\right)\frac{1}{2}\left(\mathbf{v}_i - \mathbf{v}_k\right) + \mathbf{v}_k \quad , \quad [30]$$

where $\mathbf{v}_{mci}$ = contracted position of vertex *i* toward the low point (k), and $\mathbf{v}_k$ = position of the low point.

f. Reflection and multiple contraction (Fig. 2f): multi-dimensional contractions of the vertices toward the low point after reflection, or

$$\mathbf{v}_j \Leftarrow \mathbf{v}_r$$

$$\mathbf{v}_{rmci} = \left(1 - \delta_{ik}\right)\frac{1}{2}\left(\mathbf{v}_i - \mathbf{v}_k\right) + \mathbf{v}_k \quad [31]$$

where $\mathbf{v}_{rmci}$ = reflected and contracted position of vertex *i* toward the low point (k).

Through the different simplex manipulations described above, the method approaches to the 'valley floor' and provides minimum of the cost function and location of the hip joint center.

See Press et al. (1986) for details of the downhil simplex method and the sample function **Amoeba**.

The iterations can be stopped if the change in the function value is fractionally smaller than a given tolerance:

$$\frac{|U(\mathbf{v}_j)-U(\mathbf{v}_k)|}{\left(\dfrac{|U(\mathbf{v}_j)|+|U(\mathbf{v}_k)|}{2}\right)}<TOL \quad , \quad \textbf{[32]}$$

where j = high point, k = low point, and U = cost function.

It is customary to start the iteration once again w/ the low point obtained from the previous session being one of the starting vertices to make sure that the converged low point is the true solution.

This method is based on a simple geometric relationship between the marker positions at two different instants.

If the pelvis is stationary, the thigh markers always lie on the spheres they form with the hip joint being the center.

In this case the line connecting two different positions of the same marker at two different instants is always perpendicular to the line drawn from the hip joint to their midpoint (Fig.3):

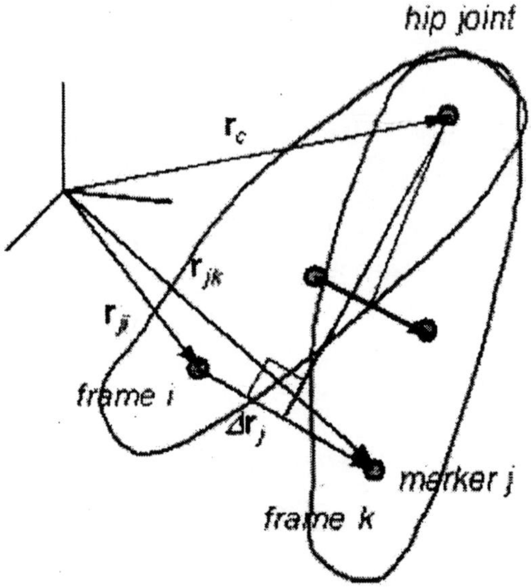

Fig. 3

$$\left(\mathbf{r}_{jk}-\mathbf{r}_{ji}\right)\cdot\left(\frac{\mathbf{r}_{jk}+\mathbf{r}_{ji}}{2}-\mathbf{r}_c\right)=0 \qquad [33]$$

The error function ε_{ji} is then

$$\varepsilon_j=\left(\mathbf{r}_{jk}-\mathbf{r}_{ji}\right)\cdot\left(\frac{\mathbf{r}_{jk}+\mathbf{r}_{ji}}{2}-\mathbf{r}_c\right) \qquad [34]$$

Let the cost function U be

$$U_{jk}=\sum_{j=1}^{m}\left[\left(\mathbf{r}_{jk}-\mathbf{r}_{ji}\right)\cdot\left(\frac{\mathbf{r}_{jk}+\mathbf{r}_{ji}}{2}-\mathbf{r}_c\right)\right]^2, \qquad [35]$$

which needs to be minimized. Minimization of the cost function U shown above has two meanings: (a) keep the angle between the two vector as close to 90 degrees as possible, and (b) keep the magnitude of the vector drawn from the joint center to the midpoint as small as possible. From [33]:

$$\left(\mathbf{r}_{jk}-\mathbf{r}_{ji}\right)\cdot\mathbf{r}_{c}=\left(\mathbf{r}_{jk}-\mathbf{r}_{ji}\right)\cdot\left(\frac{\mathbf{r}_{jk}+\mathbf{r}_{ji}}{2}\right) \quad [36]$$

Covert [36] to the equivalent matrix form:

$$\left\{\mathbf{r}_{jk}-\mathbf{r}_{ji}\right\}^{t}\cdot\left\{\mathbf{r}_{c}\right\}=\left\{\mathbf{r}_{jk}-\mathbf{r}_{ji}\right\}^{t}\cdot\left\{\frac{\mathbf{r}_{jk}+\mathbf{r}_{ji}}{2}\right\}, \quad [37]$$

where {} = column matrix operator. Expand [37] to *m* markers:

$$\mathbf{A}_{ik}\cdot\left\{\mathbf{r}_{c}\right\}=\mathbf{B}_{ik}, \quad [38]$$

where,

$$\mathbf{A}_{jk}=\begin{bmatrix} x_{1k}-x_{1i} & y_{1k}-y_{1i} & z_{1k}-z_{1i} \\ \cdot & \cdot & \cdot \\ x_{jk}-x_{ji} & y_{jk}-y_{ji} & z_{jk}-z_{ji} \\ \cdot & \cdot & \cdot \\ x_{mk}-x_{mi} & y_{mk}-y_{mi} & z_{mk}-z_{mi} \end{bmatrix}, \quad [39]$$

and

$$\mathbf{B}_{ik} = \frac{1}{2}\begin{bmatrix} \left(x_{1k}^2 + y_{1k}^2 + z_{1k}^2\right) - \left(x_{1i}^2 + y_{1i}^2 + z_{1i}^2\right) \\ \left(x_{jk}^2 + y_{jk}^2 + z_{jk}^2\right) - \left(x_{ji}^2 + y_{ji}^2 + z_{ji}^2\right) \\ \left(x_{mk}^2 + y_{mk}^2 + z_{mk}^2\right) - \left(x_{mi}^2 + y_{mi}^2 + z_{mi}^2\right) \end{bmatrix} \quad [40]$$

Form [38]:

$$\mathbf{A}_{ik}{}^{t} \cdot \mathbf{A}_{ik} \cdot \{\mathbf{r}_c\} = \mathbf{A}_{ik}{}^{t} \cdot \mathbf{B}_{ik}$$

$$\{\mathbf{r}_c\} = \left(\mathbf{A}_{ik}{}^{t} \cdot \mathbf{A}_{ik}\right)^{-1} \cdot \left(\mathbf{A}_{ik}{}^{t} \cdot \mathbf{B}_{ik}\right) \quad [41]$$

Theoretically, [41] can be expanded to multiple two-frame combinations to increase the redundancy. One issue in this method is to determine the frames to be used in the computation.

Newton's Method

For a given marker, let the random error function ε_{ji} for marker *j* at frame *i* be

$$\varepsilon_{ji}\left(\mathbf{r}_c, R_j\right) = \sqrt{\left(\mathbf{r}_c - \mathbf{r}_{ji}\right) \cdot \left(\mathbf{r}_c - \mathbf{r}_{ji}\right)} - R_j \approx 0 \quad [42]$$

For *n* frames and *m* markers, we will have a nonlinear system of *m* x *n* equations. The partial derivatives of function ε_{ji} are

$$\frac{\partial \varepsilon_{ji}}{\partial \mathbf{r}_c} = \frac{1}{\sqrt{(\mathbf{r}_c - \mathbf{r}_{ji}) \cdot (\mathbf{r}_c - \mathbf{r}_{ji})}} (\mathbf{r}_c - \mathbf{r}_{ji}) = \frac{1}{r_{ji}} (\mathbf{r}_c - \mathbf{r}_{ji})$$

$$\frac{\partial \varepsilon_{ji}}{\partial R_k} = \begin{cases} -1 & (j = k) \\ 0 & (j \neq k) \end{cases} , \quad [43]$$

where

$$r_{ji} = \sqrt{(\mathbf{r}_c - \mathbf{r}_{ji}) \cdot (\mathbf{r}_c - \mathbf{r}_{ji})}$$
$$= \sqrt{(x_c - x_{ji})^2 + (y_c - y_{ji})^2 + (z_c - z_{ji})^2} \quad [44]$$

Therefore, the **Jacobian** matrix of the nonlinear system of equations of interest can be written as

$$\mathbf{J}(\mathbf{r}_c) = \begin{bmatrix} \frac{x_c - x_{11}}{r_{11}} & \frac{y_c - y_{11}}{r_{11}} & \frac{z_c - z_{11}}{r_{11}} & -1 & \cdot & 0 & \cdot & 0 \\ \cdot & \cdot & \cdot & \cdot & \cdot & \cdot & \cdot & \cdot \\ \frac{x_c - x_{ji}}{r_{ji}} & \frac{y_c - y_{ji}}{r_{ji}} & \frac{z_c - z_{ji}}{r_{ji}} & 0 & \cdot & -1 & \cdot & 0 \\ \cdot & \cdot & \cdot & \cdot & \cdot & \cdot & \cdot & \cdot \\ \frac{x_c - x_{mn}}{r_{mn}} & \frac{y_c - y_{mn}}{r_{mn}} & \frac{z_c - z_{mn}}{r_{mn}} & 0 & \cdot & 0 & \cdot & -1 \end{bmatrix}$$

[45]

The Newton's method involves iterations and each iteration consists of three steps. The first step is to solve the following linear system of equations:

$$\mathbf{J}\left(\mathbf{r}_c^{(k-1)}\right)\begin{bmatrix}\Delta x_c\\ \Delta y_c\\ \Delta z_c\\ \Delta R_1\\ \vdots\\ \Delta R_j\\ \vdots\\ \Delta R_m\end{bmatrix}=\mathbf{E}\left(\mathbf{r}_c^{(k-1)},R_1^{(k-1)},\ldots,R_m^{(k-1)}\right)$$

$$\begin{bmatrix}\Delta x_c\\ \Delta y_c\\ \Delta z_c\\ \Delta R_1\\ \vdots\\ \Delta R_j\\ \vdots\\ \Delta R_m\end{bmatrix}=\left[\mathbf{J}\left(\mathbf{r}_c^{(k-1)}\right)^t\cdot\mathbf{J}\left(\mathbf{r}_c^{(k-1)}\right)\right]^{-1}\left[\mathbf{J}\left(\mathbf{r}_c^{(k-1)}\right)^t\cdot\mathbf{E}\left(\mathbf{r}_c^{(k-1)},R_1^{(k-1)},\ldots,R_m^{(k-1)}\right)\right]$$

, **[46]**

where, k = the current iterat on,

$\left[x_c^{(k-1)} \quad y_c^{(k-1)} \quad z_c^{(k-1)} \quad R_1^{(k-1)} \quad \ldots \quad R_j^{(k-1)} \quad \ldots \quad R_m^{(k-1)}\right]^t$ =

the solution from the previous iteration,

$$\mathbf{J}\left(\mathbf{r}_c^{(k-1)}\right)=\begin{bmatrix} \frac{x_c^{(k-1)}-x_{11}}{r_{11}} & \frac{y_c^{(k-1)}-y_{11}}{r_{11}} & \frac{z_c^{(k-1)}-z_{11}}{r_{11}} & -1 & \cdot & 0 & \cdot & 0 \\ \cdot & \cdot & \cdot & \cdot & \cdot & \cdot & \cdot & \cdot \\ \frac{x_c^{(k-1)}-x_{ji}}{r_{ji}} & \frac{y_c^{(k-1)}-y_{ji}}{r_{ji}} & \frac{z_c^{(k-1)}-z_{ji}}{r_{ji}} & 0 & \cdot & -1 & \cdot & 0 \\ \cdot & \cdot & \cdot & \cdot & \cdot & \cdot & \cdot & \cdot \\ \frac{x_c^{(k-1)}-x_{mn}}{r_{mn}} & \frac{y_c^{(k-1)}-y_{mn}}{r_{mn}} & \frac{z_c^{(k-1)}-z_{mn}}{r_{mn}} & 0 & \cdot & 0 & \cdot & -1 \end{bmatrix}$$

, **[47]**

and

$$\mathbf{B}\left(\mathbf{r}_c^{(k-1)},R_1^{(k-1)},\ldots,R_m^{(k-1)}\right)=\begin{bmatrix} -\varepsilon_{11}\left(\mathbf{r}_c^{(k-1)},R_1^{(k-1)},\ldots,R_m^{(k-1)}\right) \\ \cdot \\ -\varepsilon_{ji}\left(\mathbf{r}_c^{(k-1)},R_1^{(k-1)},\ldots,R_m^{(k-1)}\right) \\ \cdot \\ -\varepsilon_{mn}\left(\mathbf{r}_c^{(k-1)},R_1^{(k-1)},\ldots,R_m^{(k-1)}\right) \end{bmatrix}$$

[48]

In order for [46] to work, the initial guess of $\mathbf{r}_c$ and R_j's, $\begin{bmatrix} x_c^{(0)} & y_c^{(0)} & z_c^{(0)} & R_1^{(0)} & \cdot & R_j^{(0)} & \cdot & R_m^{(0)} \end{bmatrix}^t$, must be provided. The mean coordinates of the marker may be used as the initial value.

The second step in each iteration is to update $\mathbf{r}_c$ and R_j's using the solution obtained in the previous step:

$$\begin{bmatrix} x_c^{(k)} \\ y_c^{(k)} \\ z_c^{(k)} \\ R_1^{(k)} \\ \cdot \\ R_j^{(k)} \\ \cdot \\ R_m^{(k)} \end{bmatrix} = \begin{bmatrix} x_c^{(k-1)} \\ y_c^{(k-1)} \\ z_c^{(k-1)} \\ R_1^{(k-1)} \\ \cdot \\ R_j^{(k-1)} \\ \cdot \\ R_m^{(k-1)} \end{bmatrix} + \begin{bmatrix} \Delta x_c \\ \Delta y_c \\ \Delta z_c \\ \Delta R_1 \\ \cdot \\ \Delta R_j \\ \cdot \\ \Delta R_m \end{bmatrix} \quad [49]$$

The last step is to check if the solution is sufficiently converged:

$$\Delta x_c, \Delta y_c, \Delta z_c, \Delta R_1, \ldots, \Delta R_m < TOL, \quad [50]$$

where *TOL* = tolerance. The iteration will stop if the solution is sufficiently converged.

Simple Linear Method

Acknowledgement: *This method was suggested by* ***Dr. Yong-San Yoon*** *of Korea Advanced Institute of Science and Technology (KAIST)*

From [1]:

$$\begin{aligned} 0 &= (\mathbf{r}_{ji} - \mathbf{r}_c)\cdot(\mathbf{r}_{ji} - \mathbf{r}_c) - R_j^2 \\ &= \mathbf{r}_{ji}\cdot\mathbf{r}_{ji} - 2\mathbf{r}_{ji}\cdot\mathbf{r}_c + \mathbf{r}_c\cdot\mathbf{r}_c - R_j^2 \end{aligned} \quad [51]$$

[51] can be rewritten as

$$2\mathbf{r}_{ji}\cdot\mathbf{r}_c + P_j = \mathbf{r}_{ji}\cdot\mathbf{r}_{ji}, \quad [52]$$

where

$$P_j = R_j^2 - \mathbf{r}_c\cdot\mathbf{r}_c. \quad [53]$$

[52] is basically a linear equation of $\mathbf{r}_c$ and P_j. Expand [52] to *n* frames and *m* markers to obtain

$$\begin{bmatrix} 2x_{11} & 2y_{11} & 2z_{11} & 1 & \cdot & 0 & \cdot & 0 \\ \cdot & \cdot & \cdot & \cdot & \cdot & \cdot & \cdot & \cdot \\ 2x_{ji} & 2y_{ji} & 2z_{ji} & 0 & \cdot & 1 & \cdot & 0 \\ \cdot & \cdot & \cdot & \cdot & \cdot & \cdot & \cdot & \cdot \\ 2x_{mn} & 2y_{mn} & 2z_{mn} & 0 & \cdot & 0 & \cdot & 1 \end{bmatrix} \begin{bmatrix} x_c \\ y_c \\ z_c \\ P_1 \\ \cdot \\ P_j \\ \cdot \\ P_m \end{bmatrix} = \begin{bmatrix} x_{11}^2 + y_{11}^2 + z_{11}^2 \\ \cdot \\ x_{ji}^2 + y_{ji}^2 + z_{ji}^2 \\ \cdot \\ x_{mn}^2 + y_{mn}^2 + z_{mn}^2 \end{bmatrix}$$

[54]

Use the typical least square approach to solve the system of equations. R_j's of the markers can be computed afterward using [53], if necessary.

Computation of a Rotation Matrix

Rotation of a Body

In motion analysis, it is often necessary to compute the transformation matrix directly from the coordinates of the markers fixed on a moving body. This can be done if more than 3 markers are fixed on the body. Once the transformation matrix is known, the orientation angles and eventually the location of center of rotation as well may be computed.

As shown in Figure 1, an object rotates from position 1 to position 2 about the center of rotation (*C*). Let rotation matrix **R** be

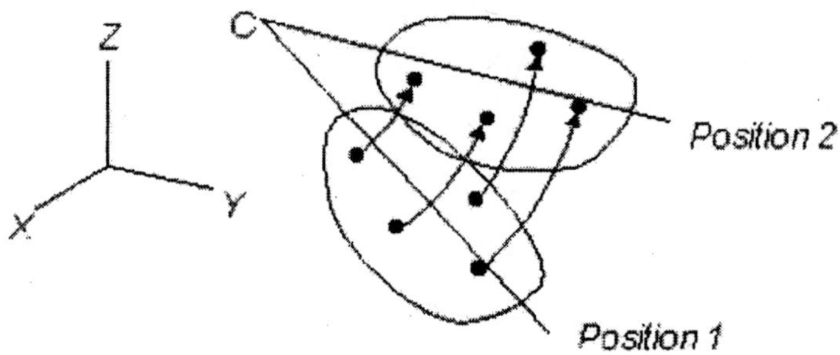

Figure 1

$$\mathbf{R} = \begin{bmatrix} r_{11} & r_{12} & r_{13} \\ r_{21} & r_{22} & r_{23} \\ r_{31} & r_{32} & r_{33} \end{bmatrix} \quad [1]$$

The following relationship holds:

$$\begin{bmatrix} x_{2i} - x_c \\ y_{2i} - y_c \\ z_{2i} - z_c \end{bmatrix} = \begin{bmatrix} r_{11} & r_{12} & r_{13} \\ r_{21} & r_{22} & r_{23} \\ r_{31} & r_{32} & r_{33} \end{bmatrix} \begin{bmatrix} x_{1i} - x_c \\ y_{1i} - y_c \\ z_{1i} - z_c \end{bmatrix}$$

$$\mathbf{x}_{2i} - \mathbf{x}_c = \mathbf{R}(\mathbf{x}_{1i} - \mathbf{x}_c) \quad , \quad [2]$$

where $[x_c, y_c, z_c]$ = the coordinates of the center of rotation, $[x_{1i}, y_{1i}, z_{1i}]$ = the position of marker *i* at position 1, and $[x_{2i}, y_{2i}, z_{2i}]$ = the position of marker *i* at position 2. [2] involves a total of 12 unknowns, thus requires at least 4 markers since each marker provides 3 equations.

In an effort to reduce the number of unknowns involved, [2] can be reduced to

$$\begin{bmatrix} x_{2i} - \bar{x}_2 \\ y_{2i} - \bar{y}_2 \\ z_{2i} - \bar{z}_2 \end{bmatrix} = \begin{bmatrix} r_{11} & r_{12} & r_{13} \\ r_{21} & r_{22} & r_{23} \\ r_{31} & r_{32} & r_{33} \end{bmatrix} \begin{bmatrix} x_{1i} - \bar{x}_1 \\ y_{1i} - \bar{y}_1 \\ z_{1i} - \bar{z}_1 \end{bmatrix}$$

$$\begin{bmatrix} x'_{2i} \\ y'_{2i} \\ z'_{2i} \end{bmatrix} = \begin{bmatrix} r_{11} & r_{12} & r_{13} \\ r_{21} & r_{22} & r_{23} \\ r_{31} & r_{32} & r_{33} \end{bmatrix} \begin{bmatrix} x'_{1i} \\ y'_{1i} \\ z'_{1i} \end{bmatrix}$$

$$\mathbf{x}'_{2i} = \mathbf{R}\mathbf{x}'_{1i} \,, \qquad \textbf{[3]}$$

where

$$\bar{x} = \frac{\sum_i x_i}{N} \quad \bar{y} = \frac{\sum_i y_i}{N} \quad \bar{z} = \frac{\sum_i z_i}{N} \qquad \textbf{[4]}$$

$$\mathbf{x}'_i = \begin{bmatrix} x_i - \bar{x} & y_i - \bar{y} & z_i - \bar{z} \end{bmatrix}^t \,, \qquad \textbf{[5]}$$

and N = number of markers. [3] basically shows the rotational transformation about the mean-coordinate point within the body, involving 9 unknowns. At least 3 markers are required here. From [3]:

$$\mathbf{x}'_{2i} - \mathbf{R}\mathbf{x}'_{1i} = 0 \qquad \textbf{[6]}$$

The Least-Square Approach

Applying the least-square approach to [6]:

$$\frac{1}{N}\sum_{i=1}^{N} (\mathbf{x}'_{2i} - \mathbf{R}\mathbf{x}'_{1i})^t (\mathbf{x}'_{2i} - \mathbf{R}\mathbf{x}'_{1i}) \Rightarrow \min \qquad \textbf{[7]}$$

Further developing [7]:

$$\frac{1}{N}\sum_{i=1}^{N}(\mathbf{x'}_{2i}-\mathbf{Rx'}_{1i})^t(\mathbf{x'}_{2i}-\mathbf{Rx'}_{1i})$$
$$=\frac{1}{N}\sum_{i=1}^{N}\left[\mathbf{x'}_{2i}{}^t\,\mathbf{x'}_{2i}-\mathbf{x'}_{2i}{}^t(\mathbf{Rx'}_{1i})-(\mathbf{Rx'}_{1i})^t\mathbf{x'}_{2i}+(\mathbf{Rx'}_{1i})^t(\mathbf{Rx'}_{1i})\right]$$
$$=\frac{1}{N}\sum_{i=1}^{N}\left[\mathbf{x'}_{2i}{}^t\,\mathbf{x'}_{2i}-\mathbf{x'}_{2i}{}^t\,\mathbf{Rx'}_{1i}-\left(\mathbf{x'}_{2i}{}^t\,\mathbf{Rx'}_{1i}\right)^t+\mathbf{x'}_{1i}{}^t\,\mathbf{x'}_{1i}\right]$$
$$=\frac{1}{N}\sum_{i=1}^{N}\left(\mathbf{x'}_{2i}{}^t\,\mathbf{x'}_{2i}-2\mathbf{x'}_{2i}{}^t\,\mathbf{Rx'}_{1i}+\mathbf{x'}_{1i}{}^t\,\mathbf{x'}_{1i}\right)$$
$$=\frac{1}{N}\sum_{i=1}^{N}\mathbf{x'}_{2i}{}^t\,\mathbf{x'}_{2i}-\frac{2}{N}\sum_{i=1}^{N}\mathbf{x'}_{2i}{}^t\,\mathbf{Rx'}_{1i}+\frac{1}{N}\sum_{i=1}^{N}\mathbf{x'}_{1i}{}^t\,\mathbf{x'}_{1i}. \quad [8]$$

since

$$(\mathbf{Rx'}_{1i})^t(\mathbf{Rx'}_{1i})=\mathbf{x'}_{1i}{}^t\,\mathbf{R}^t\mathbf{Rx'}_{1i}$$
$$=\mathbf{x'}_{1i}{}^t\left(\mathbf{R}^t\mathbf{R}\right)\mathbf{x'}_{1i}$$
$$=\mathbf{x'}_{1i}{}^t\,\mathbf{x'}_{1i}. \quad [9]$$

and

$$\left(\mathbf{x'}_{2i}{}^t\,\mathbf{Rx'}_{1i}\right)^t=\mathbf{x'}_{2i}{}^t\,\mathbf{Rx'}_{1i}. \quad [10]$$

Matrix $\mathbf{x'}_{2i}{}^t\,\mathbf{Rx'}_{1i}$ shown in [10] is a 1 x 1 matrix (scalar) so it is equal to its transpose.

The least-square approach presented in [7] is in fact equivalent to

$$\frac{1}{N}\sum_{i=1}^{N}\mathbf{x'}_{2i}{}^t\,\mathbf{Rx'}_{1i}\Rightarrow\max. \quad [11]$$

Further developing [11]:

$$\frac{1}{N}\sum_{i=1}^{N}\mathbf{x'}_{2i}{}^{t}\mathbf{R}\mathbf{x'}_{1i} = \frac{1}{N}\sum_{i=1}^{N}\begin{bmatrix} x'_{2i} & y'_{2i} & z'_{2i}\end{bmatrix}\begin{bmatrix} r_{11} & r_{12} & r_{13} \\ r_{21} & r_{22} & r_{23} \\ r_{31} & r_{32} & r_{33}\end{bmatrix}\begin{bmatrix} x'_{1i} \\ y'_{1i} \\ z'_{1i}\end{bmatrix}$$

$$= \frac{1}{N}\sum_{i=1}^{N}\begin{bmatrix} x'_{2i} & y'_{2i} & z'_{2i}\end{bmatrix}\begin{bmatrix} r_{11}x'_{1i}+r_{12}y'_{1i}+r_{13}z'_{1i} \\ r_{21}x'_{1i}+r_{22}y'_{1i}+r_{23}z'_{1i} \\ r_{31}x'_{1i}+r_{32}y'_{1i}+r_{33}z'_{1i}\end{bmatrix}$$

$$= \frac{1}{N}\sum_{i=1}^{N}\Big[x'_{2i}\left(r_{11}x'_{1i}+r_{12}y'_{1i}+r_{13}z'_{1i}\right)+y'_{2i}\left(r_{21}x'_{1i}+r_{22}y'_{1i}+r_{23}z'_{1i}\right)$$

$$+z'_{2i}\left(r_{31}x'_{1i}+r_{32}y'_{1i}+r_{33}z'_{1i}\right)\Big]$$

$$= \frac{1}{N}\sum_{i=1}^{N}tr\left(\mathbf{R}^{t}\mathbf{x'}_{2i}\,\mathbf{x'}_{1i}{}^{t}\right)$$

$$= tr\left(\mathbf{R}^{t}\frac{1}{N}\sum_{i=1}^{N}\mathbf{x'}_{2i}\,\mathbf{x'}_{1i}{}^{t}\right).$$

[12]

since

$$\mathbf{R}^{t}\mathbf{x'}_{2i}\,\mathbf{x'}_{1i}{}^{t} = \begin{bmatrix} r_{11} & r_{21} & r_{31} \\ r_{12} & r_{22} & r_{32} \\ r_{13} & r_{23} & r_{33}\end{bmatrix}\begin{bmatrix} x_{2i} \\ y_{2i} \\ z_{2i}\end{bmatrix}\begin{bmatrix} x_{1i} & y_{1i} & z_{1i}\end{bmatrix}$$

$$= \begin{bmatrix} r_{11} & r_{21} & r_{31} \\ r_{12} & r_{22} & r_{32} \\ r_{13} & r_{23} & r_{33}\end{bmatrix}\begin{bmatrix} x_{2i}x_{1i} & x_{2i}y_{1i} & x_{2i}z_{1i} \\ y_{2i}x_{1i} & y_{2i}y_{1i} & y_{2i}z_{1i} \\ z_{2i}x_{1i} & z_{2i}y_{1i} & z_{2i}z_{1i}\end{bmatrix}$$

$$= \begin{bmatrix} r_{11}x_{2i}x_{1i}+r_{21}y_{2i}x_{1i}+r_{31}z_{2i}x_{1i} & & \\ & r_{12}x_{2i}y_{1i}+r_{22}y_{2i}y_{1i}+r_{32}z_{2i}y_{1i} & \\ & & r_{13}x_{2i}z_{1i}+r_{23}y_{2i}z_{1i}+r_{33}z_{2i}z_{1i}\end{bmatrix},$$

[13]

where $tr(\mathbf{a})$ = the trace (sum of the diagonal terms) of matrix **a**.

Now, let

$$\mathbf{c} \equiv \frac{1}{N}\sum_{i=1}^{N} \mathbf{x}'_{2i}\,\mathbf{x}'_{1i}{}^{t} \quad , \quad [14]$$

where **c** = **the cross-dispersion matrix** or **the correlation matrix**.

From [11], [12] & [14]:

$$tr\left(\mathbf{R}^{t}\mathbf{c}\right) \Rightarrow \max \quad [15]$$

Computation of the Rotation Matrix

The singular value decomposition of matrix c shown in [15] provides

$$\mathbf{c} = \mathbf{u} \cdot \mathbf{w} \cdot \mathbf{v}^{t} , \quad [16]$$

where **u** & **v** = orthogonal matrices, and **w** = diagonal matrix containing the singular values of **c**. See the Singular Value Decomposition page in this section for the details of this method. Substituting [16] into [15],

$$\begin{aligned} tr\left(\mathbf{R}^{t}\mathbf{u}\mathbf{w}\mathbf{v}^{t}\right) &= tr\left(\mathbf{v}^{t}\mathbf{R}^{t}\mathbf{u}\mathbf{w}\right) \\ &= tr\left\{\left(\mathbf{v}^{t}\mathbf{R}^{t}\mathbf{u}\right)\mathbf{w}\right\} \\ &= tr\left(\mathbf{c}'\mathbf{w}\right) \Rightarrow \max , \quad [17] \end{aligned}$$

where

$$\mathbf{c}' = \mathbf{v}^{t}\mathbf{R}^{t}\mathbf{u} , \quad [18]$$

since

$$tr(\mathbf{ab}) = tr\left\{\begin{bmatrix} a_{11} & a_{12} & a_{13} \\ a_{21} & a_{22} & a_{23} \\ a_{31} & a_{32} & a_{33} \end{bmatrix}\begin{bmatrix} b_{11} & b_{12} & b_{13} \\ b_{21} & b_{22} & b_{23} \\ b_{31} & b_{32} & b_{33} \end{bmatrix}\right\}$$

$$= tr\left\{\begin{bmatrix} a_{11}b_{11} + a_{12}b_{21} + a_{13}b_{31} & & \\ & a_{21}b_{12} + a_{22}b_{22} + a_{23}b_{32} & \\ & & a_{31}b_{13} + a_{32}b_{23} + a_{33}b_{33} \end{bmatrix}\right\}$$

$$= a_{11}b_{11} + a_{12}b_{21} + a_{13}b_{31} + a_{21}b_{12} + a_{22}b_{22} + a_{23}b_{32} + a_{31}b_{13} + a_{32}b_{23} + a_{33}b_{33}$$

$$tr(\mathbf{ba}) = b_{11}a_{11} + b_{12}a_{21} + b_{13}a_{31} + b_{21}a_{12} + b_{22}a_{22} + b_{23}a_{32} + b_{31}a_{13} + b_{32}a_{23} + b_{33}a_{33}$$

$$= a_{11}b_{11} + a_{12}b_{21} + a_{13}b_{31} + a_{21}b_{12} + a_{22}b_{22} + a_{23}b_{32} + a_{31}b_{13} + a_{32}b_{23} + a_{33}b_{33}$$

$$tr(\mathbf{ab}) = tr(\mathbf{ba}).$$

[19]

Since matrix **w** shown in [17] is a diagonal matrix, only the diagonal elements of matrix **c'** shown in [17] and [18] can contribute to the trace.

In addition, matrix **c'** must be orthogonal because all three matrices composing **c'** are orthogonal.

Therefore, *tr*(**c'w**) becomes maximum when **c'** is the identity matrix:

$$\mathbf{v}^t\mathbf{R}^t\mathbf{u} = \mathbf{I} \quad \textbf{[20]}$$

Therefore,

$$v\left(v^tR^tu\right)u^t = vIu^t$$
$$\left(vv^t\right)R^t\left(uu^t\right) = vu^t$$
$$R^t = vu^t$$
$$R = \left(vu^t\right)^t = uv^t \qquad [21]$$

One problem that may arise here in using [21] is that matrix **R** obtained from [21] can have a determinant of -1. In other words, one can obtain a reflection matrix of the desired rotation matrix. [21] can be modified to solve this problem:

$$\mathbf{R} = \mathbf{u}\begin{bmatrix} 1 & 0 & 0 \\ 0 & 1 & 0 \\ 0 & 0 & \det\left(\mathbf{uv}^t\right) \end{bmatrix}\mathbf{v}^t \qquad [22]$$

Application

[22] can be used effectively in quantifying the joint motions. As shown in Figure 2, one can transform the global coordinates of the markers fixed to the distal segment to those described in the proximal segment's reference frame (frame *P*):

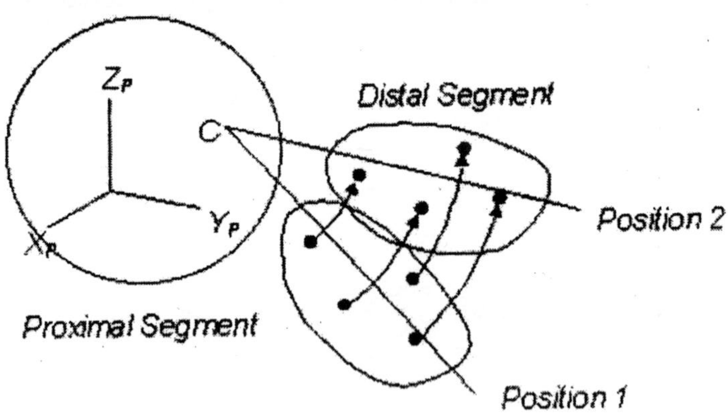

Figure 2

$$\mathbf{x}_i^{(P)} = \mathbf{T}_{P/G}(\mathbf{X}_i - \mathbf{X}_P), \quad [23]$$

where i = marker, $\mathbf{x}$ = the position of the marker observed in frame P, $\mathbf{T}_{P/G}$ = the transformation matrix from the global frame to frame P, $\mathbf{X}$ = the global position of the marker, and $\mathbf{X}_P$ = the global position of the origin of frame P. Thus, vectors $\mathbf{x}'_{1i}$ & $\mathbf{x}'_{2i}$ shown in [2] can be obtained as

$$\mathbf{x}_{1i}^{(P)} = \mathbf{T}_{P/G1}(\mathbf{X}_{1i} - \mathbf{X}_{P1})$$
$$\mathbf{x}_{2i}^{(P)} = \mathbf{T}_{P/G2}(\mathbf{X}_{2i} - \mathbf{X}_{P2}). \quad [24]$$

The rotation matrix to be obtained from [22] in this case is therefore the joint motion matrix.

One thing, at least 3 markers must be commonly observed at both positions (N shown in [7] >= 3).

Helical (Screw) Axis

The motion of an object from one position to another can be broken down into a rotation about and a translation along the instantaneous axis of rotation.

One exception will be when the object shows pure translation but no rotation. This instantaneous axis of rotation is often called **helical axis (screw axis)** (Fig. 1).

The helical axis is a useful tool to analyze the relative motion of a rigid object to another, especially the joint motion. Human body joints have varying degrees of freedom depending on the shapes of the articulating bones:

ball-and-socket (3), condyloid (2), hinge (1), and pivot (1). Degrees of freedom in a joint basically means how many axes of rotation are present in the joint. The instantaneous axis of rotation of a joint can be viewed as a helical axis and the relative translation of the bones along the instantaneous axis of rotation can be quantified along this line.

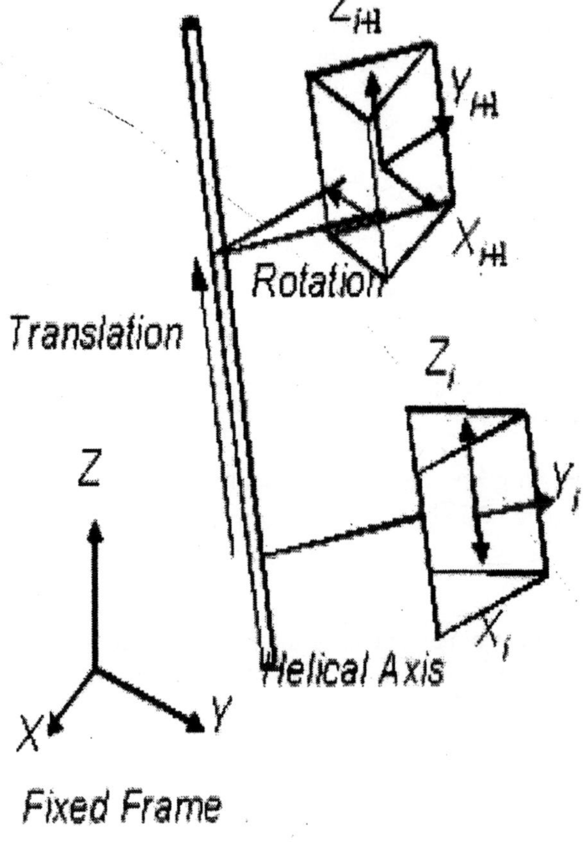

[Fig. 1]

Displacement of a Point Fixed to the Moving Body

Vector **d** shown in [Fig. 2] is the displacement of a point fixed to the moving body from position i to i+1 due to the object's rotation $\boldsymbol{\varphi}$ ($0 < \varphi < \pi$) and translation **L**.

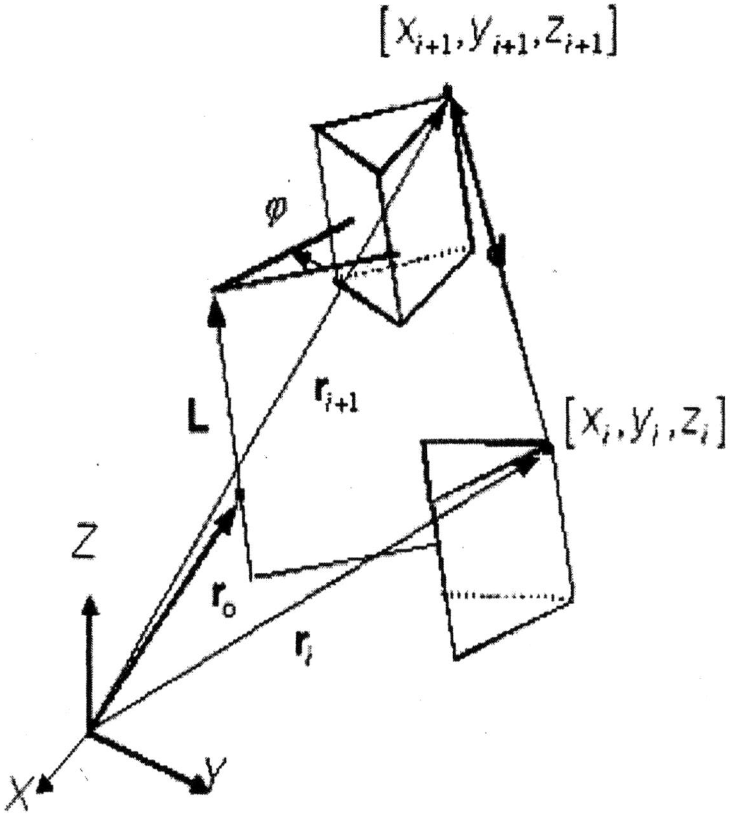

[Fig. 2]

Vector **L** shows the orientation of the helical axis:

$$\mathbf{L} = L\mathbf{n} = L\left[n_x, n_y, n_z\right], \quad [1]$$

where L = magnitude of the translation along the helical axis, and **n** = the unit vector of the helical axis. Vector $\mathbf{r}_o$ is the position vector of the helical axis. The displacement from position i to i+1 can be described as the sum of the translation along (**L**) and the displacement due to the rotation about the helical axis ($\mathbf{d}_R$) (Fig. 3):

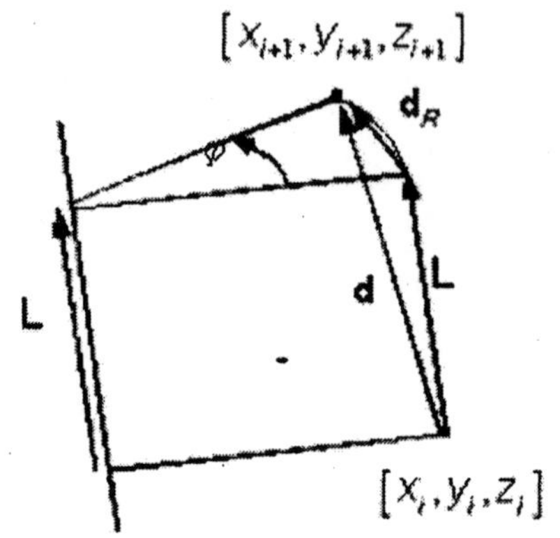

[Fig. 3]

$$\mathbf{d} = \mathbf{L} + \mathbf{d}_R. \quad [2]$$

Helical Rotation Matrix

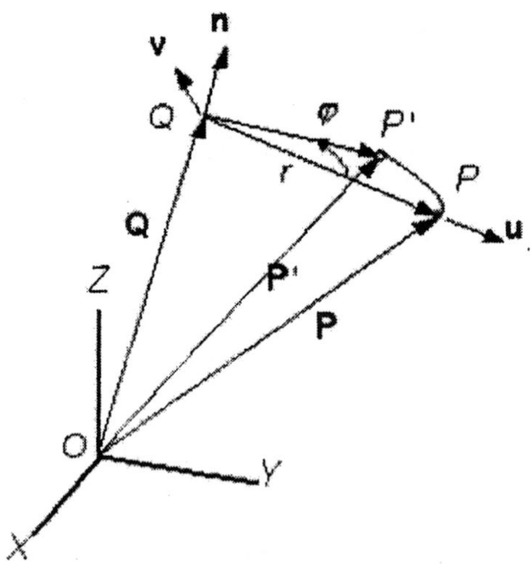

[Fig. 4]

Focus on the rotation of a point fixed to the moving body (*P* shown in [Fig. 4]) about the helical axis passing through the origin of the reference frame. **n** is the unit vector of the helical axis. *P* is rotated around **n** to *P'*. Line *QP* is the perpendicular distance from **n** to *P* and vector *QP* can be written as *r***u**, where **u** is the unit vector normal to **n**, and *r* = the radius. As vector *r***u** rotates by angle φ around **n**, *P* moves to *P'*. Vectors **Q**, **P**, and **P'** are the position vectors of points *Q*, *P*, and *P'*, respectively. Unit vector **v** (Fig. 4), normal to both **n** and **u**, can be defined as

$$\mathbf{v} = \mathbf{n} \times \mathbf{u} \qquad [3]$$

From [Fig. 4]:

$$\mathbf{P}' = \mathbf{Q} + (r \cdot \cos\varphi)\mathbf{u} + (r \cdot \sin\varphi)\mathbf{v} \quad , \quad [4]$$

and

$$r\mathbf{u} = \mathbf{P} - \mathbf{Q} \qquad [5]$$

From [3] and [5]:

$$\mathbf{v} = \mathbf{n} \times \frac{(\mathbf{P} - \mathbf{Q})}{r} \qquad [6]$$

From [4], [5], and [6]:

$$\begin{aligned} \mathbf{P}' &= \mathbf{Q} + (\mathbf{P} - \mathbf{Q})\cos\varphi + r\sin\varphi \frac{\mathbf{n} \times (\mathbf{P} - \mathbf{Q})}{r} \\ &= \mathbf{Q} + (\mathbf{P} - \mathbf{Q})\cos\varphi + \sin\varphi(\mathbf{n} \times \mathbf{P}) \\ &= \mathbf{Q}(1 - \cos\varphi) + \mathbf{P}\cos\varphi + (\mathbf{n} \times \mathbf{P})\sin\varphi \quad , \quad [7] \end{aligned}$$

since $\mathbf{n} \times \mathbf{Q} = 0$

Q is the projection of **P** on **n** or

$$\mathbf{Q} = \mathbf{n}(\mathbf{n} \cdot \mathbf{P}) \quad [8]$$

From [7] and [8]:

$$\mathbf{P}' = \mathbf{n}(\mathbf{n} \cdot \mathbf{P})(1 - \cos\varphi) + \mathbf{P}\cos\varphi + (\mathbf{n} \times \mathbf{P})\sin\varphi$$

$$\begin{aligned} \{\mathbf{P}'\} &= \{\mathbf{n}\}\{\mathbf{n}\}^t\{\mathbf{P}\}(1 - \cos\varphi) + \mathbf{1}\{\mathbf{P}\}\cos\varphi + \langle\mathbf{n}\rangle\{\mathbf{P}\}\sin\varphi \\ &= \left[(1 - \cos\varphi)\{\mathbf{n}\}\{\mathbf{n}\}^t + \cos\varphi\mathbf{1} + \sin\varphi\langle\mathbf{n}\rangle\right]\{\mathbf{P}\} \\ &= \mathbf{H}\{\mathbf{P}\} \end{aligned}$$

$$\mathbf{H} = (1 - \cos\varphi)\{\mathbf{n}\}\{\mathbf{n}\}^t + \cos\varphi\mathbf{1} + \sin\varphi\langle\mathbf{n}\rangle \quad [9]$$

where { } = column matrix operator, t = transpose, **1** = identity matrix, **H** = helical rotation matrix, and $\langle\ \rangle$ = cross product operator or

$$\langle\mathbf{n}\rangle = \begin{bmatrix} 0 & -n_z & n_y \\ n_z & 0 & -n_x \\ -n_y & n_x & 0 \end{bmatrix} \quad [10]$$

$\langle\mathbf{n}\rangle$ in [10] has the following properties among many:

$$tr\left(\langle \mathbf{n} \rangle\right) = 0$$
$$\langle \mathbf{n} \rangle^t = -\langle \mathbf{n} \rangle$$
$$\{\mathbf{n}\}^t \cdot \langle \mathbf{n} \rangle = 0$$
$$\{\mathbf{n}\}^t \cdot \langle \mathbf{n} \rangle^t = -\{\mathbf{n}\}^t \cdot \langle \mathbf{n} \rangle = 0$$
$$\langle \mathbf{n} \rangle \{\mathbf{n}\} = \left[\{\mathbf{n}\}^t \langle \mathbf{n} \rangle^t\right]^t = -\left[\{\mathbf{n}\}^t \langle \mathbf{n} \rangle\right]^t = 0$$
$$\langle \mathbf{n} \rangle^t \{\mathbf{n}\} = -\langle \mathbf{n} \rangle \{\mathbf{n}\} = 0$$
$$\langle \mathbf{n} \rangle^t \langle \mathbf{n} \rangle = \begin{bmatrix} n_y^2 + n_z^2 & -n_x n_y & -n_x n_z \\ -n_y n_x & n_z^2 + n_x^2 & -n_y n_z \\ -n_z n_x & -n_z n_y & n_x^2 + n_y^2 \end{bmatrix} = \mathbf{1} - \{\mathbf{n}\}\{\mathbf{n}\}^t$$
$$tr\left(\langle \mathbf{n} \rangle^t \langle \mathbf{n} \rangle\right) = tr(\mathbf{1}) - tr\left(\{\mathbf{n}\}\{\mathbf{n}\}^t\right) = 2$$
$$\langle \mathbf{n} \rangle^t \langle \mathbf{n} \rangle = -\langle \mathbf{n} \rangle \langle \mathbf{n} \rangle = \langle \mathbf{n} \rangle \langle \mathbf{n} \rangle^t$$

, **[11]**

where

$$\{\mathbf{n}\}^t \{\mathbf{n}\} = 1$$
$$\{\mathbf{n}\}\{\mathbf{n}\}^t = \begin{bmatrix} n_x^2 & n_x n_y & n_x n_z \\ n_y n_x & n_y^2 & n_y n_z \\ n_z n_x & n_z n_y & n_z^2 \end{bmatrix}$$
$$tr\left(\{\mathbf{n}\}\{\mathbf{n}\}^t\right) = 1$$

[12]

tr() in [12] is the sum of the diagonal terms or the **trace** of the matrix. Remember here that both **P** and **P**' in [7] are described in the *XYZ*-system and **H** is thus a rotation matrix, not a transformation matrix. [11] is the general form of the rotation matrix about an arbitrary axis of rotation that passes through the origin of the reference frame.

Solutions

Now, let's get back to the original problem illustrated in [Fig. 2]. Let the position of the helical axis, $\mathbf{r}_o$, be

$$\mathbf{r}_o = [x_o, y_o, z_o] \quad [13]$$

From [9], and [2] and [Fig. 2]:

$$\{\mathbf{r}_{i+1,j} - \mathbf{r}_o\} = \mathbf{H}\{\mathbf{r}_{i,j} - \mathbf{r}_o\} + \{\mathbf{L}\}, \quad [14]$$

where i = frame, and j = marker. Expand [14] for N markers and take the mean:

$$\frac{1}{N}\sum_{j=1}^{N}\{\mathbf{r}_{i+1,j} - \mathbf{r}_o\} = \frac{1}{N}\sum_{j=1}^{N}\left[\mathbf{H}\{\mathbf{r}_{i,j} - \mathbf{r}_o\} + \{\mathbf{L}\}\right]$$

$$\{\bar{\mathbf{r}}_{i+1} - \mathbf{r}_o\} = \mathbf{H}\{\bar{\mathbf{r}}_i - \mathbf{r}_o\} + \{\mathbf{L}\}, \quad [15]$$

where $\bar{\mathbf{r}}_i$ = mean position of the markers in frame i, etc. Modify [14] using the mean position vector and apply [15]:

$$\mathbf{r}_{i,j} = \mathbf{x}_{i,j} + \bar{\mathbf{r}}_i$$

$$\mathbf{r}_{i+1,j} = \mathbf{x}_{i+1,j} + \bar{\mathbf{r}}_{i+1}$$

$$\{\mathbf{x}_{i+1,j} + \bar{\mathbf{r}}_{i+1} - \mathbf{r}_o\} = \mathbf{H}\{\mathbf{x}_{i,j} + \bar{\mathbf{r}}_i - \mathbf{r}_o\} + \{\mathbf{L}\}$$

$$\{\mathbf{x}_{i+1,j}\} + \{\bar{\mathbf{r}}_{i+1} - \mathbf{r}_o\} = \mathbf{H}\{\mathbf{x}_{i,j}\} + \mathbf{H}\{\bar{\mathbf{r}}_i - \mathbf{r}_o\} + \{\mathbf{L}\}$$

$$\{\mathbf{x}_{i+1,j}\} = \mathbf{H}\{\mathbf{x}_{i,j}\}, \quad [16]$$

where $\mathbf{x}_{i,j}$ = the relative position of marker j to the mean position ($\bar{\mathbf{r}}_i$) in frame i, etc. In other words, **H** can be computed directly from the coordinates of the markers attached to the rotating body. This operation is independent from the translation along the helical axis (**L**). See the Computation of the Rotation Matrix page and the Singular Value Decomposition (SVD) page for details on how to compute the rotation matrix based on the least square method and singular value decomposition.

From [14]:

$$\begin{aligned}\{\mathbf{r}_{i+1,j}\} &= \mathbf{H}\{\mathbf{r}_{i,j}\} + (\mathbf{1}-\mathbf{H})\{\mathbf{r}_o\} + \{\mathbf{L}\} \\ &= \mathbf{H}\{\mathbf{r}_{i,j}\} + \{\mathbf{t}\}\end{aligned} \quad , \quad [17]$$

where

$$\{\mathbf{t}\} = (\mathbf{1}-\mathbf{H})\{\mathbf{r}_o\} + \{\mathbf{L}\} = (\mathbf{1}-\mathbf{H})\{\mathbf{r}_o\} + L\{\mathbf{n}\} \quad . \quad [18]$$

t is constant for all markers. Expand [17] for N markers and compute the mean:

$$\begin{aligned}\{\mathbf{t}\} &= \{\mathbf{r}_{i+1,j}\} - \mathbf{H}\{\mathbf{r}_{i,j}\} \\ \frac{1}{N}\sum_{j=1}^{N}\{\mathbf{t}\} &= \frac{1}{N}\sum_{j=1}^{N}\left[\{\mathbf{r}_{i+1,j}\} - \mathbf{H}\{\mathbf{r}_{i,j}\}\right] \\ \{\mathbf{t}\} &= \{\bar{\mathbf{r}}_{i+1}\} - \mathbf{H}\{\bar{\mathbf{r}}_i\}\end{aligned} \quad [19]$$

Once **H** is known, **t** can be computed using [19].

Now, both **H** and **t** are known and from [9] and [11]:

$$tr\,(\mathbf{H}) = (1-\cos\varphi)\cdot tr\left(\{\mathbf{n}\}\{\mathbf{n}\}^t\right) + \cos\varphi\cdot tr\,(\mathbf{1}) + \sin\varphi\cdot tr\,(\langle\mathbf{n}\rangle)$$
$$= 1 + 2\cos\varphi$$
$$\cos\varphi = \frac{tr\,(\mathbf{H})-1}{2}$$
$$\varphi = \cos^{-1}\left[\frac{tr\,(\mathbf{H})-1}{2}\right] \qquad (0<\varphi<\pi)$$

[20]

Angle $\varphi\,(0<\varphi<\pi)$ can be obtained from [20]. Remember here that angle φ can not be negative. If the rotation happens in the opposite direction, vector **n** must be reversed while angle φ still maintains a positive value. Also from [9]:

$$\mathbf{H}^t = (1-\cos\varphi)\{\mathbf{n}\}\{\mathbf{n}\}^t + \cos\varphi\mathbf{1} + \sin\varphi\langle\mathbf{n}\rangle^t$$
$$= (1-\cos\varphi)\{\mathbf{n}\}\{\mathbf{n}\}^t + \cos\varphi\mathbf{1} - \sin\varphi\langle\mathbf{n}\rangle \qquad \textbf{[21]}$$

Thus, from [9], [11], and [21]:

$$\mathbf{H}-\mathbf{H}^t = 2\sin\varphi\langle\mathbf{n}\rangle$$
$$\left(\mathbf{H}-\mathbf{H}^t\right)^t\left(\mathbf{H}-\mathbf{H}^t\right) = 4\sin^2\varphi\langle\mathbf{n}\rangle^t\langle\mathbf{n}\rangle$$
$$tr\left[\left(\mathbf{H}-\mathbf{H}^t\right)^t\left(\mathbf{H}-\mathbf{H}^t\right)\right] = 4\sin^2\varphi\cdot tr\left(\langle\mathbf{n}\rangle^t\langle\mathbf{n}\rangle\right)$$
$$tr\left[\left(\mathbf{H}-\mathbf{H}^t\right)^t\left(\mathbf{H}-\mathbf{H}^t\right)\right] = 2\left[(h_{12}-h_{21})^2+(h_{23}-h_{32})^2+(h_{31}-h_{13})^2\right]$$
$$(h_{12}-h_{21})^2+(h_{23}-h_{32})^2+(h_{31}-h_{13})^2 = 4\sin^2\varphi$$
$$\sin\varphi = \frac{1}{2}\sqrt{(h_{12}-h_{21})^2+(h_{23}-h_{32})^2+(h_{31}-h_{13})^2}$$

[22]

where

$$\mathbf{H}=\begin{bmatrix} h_{11} & h_{12} & h_{13} \\ h_{21} & h_{22} & h_{23} \\ h_{31} & h_{32} & h_{33} \end{bmatrix} \quad \textbf{[23]}$$

From [9] and [21]:

$$\frac{1}{2}\left(\mathbf{H}+\mathbf{H}^{t}\right)=(1-\cos\varphi)\{\mathbf{n}\}\{\mathbf{n}\}^{t}+\cos\varphi\mathbf{1} \quad \textbf{[24]}$$

From [24]:

$$\frac{1}{2}\left(\mathbf{H}+\mathbf{H}^{t}\right)-\cos\varphi\mathbf{1}=(1-\cos\phi)\mathbf{n}\mathbf{n}^{t}=\left[\{\mathbf{n}_1\} \quad \{\mathbf{n}_2\} \quad \{\mathbf{n}_3\}\right],$$

[25]

where $\{\mathbf{n}_1\}$, $\{\mathbf{n}_2\}$, and $\{\mathbf{n}_3\}$ = three column matrices. $\mathbf{n}_1$, $\mathbf{n}_2$ & $\mathbf{n}_3$ are all parallel to **n** since

$$\begin{aligned} k\{\mathbf{n}\}\{\mathbf{n}\}^{t} &= \left[kn_x\{\mathbf{n}\} \quad kn_y\{\mathbf{n}\} \quad kn_z\{\mathbf{n}\}\right] \\ &= \left[\{\mathbf{n}_1\} \quad \{\mathbf{n}_2\} \quad \{\mathbf{n}_3\}\right] \end{aligned} , \quad \textbf{[26]}$$

where k = a scalar. One can compute **n** from any column of the matrix shown in [25]. Use the column that gives the maximum magnitude because it is the least error-prone:

$$\mathbf{n}=\frac{1}{\left|\mathbf{n}_{max}\right|}\mathbf{n}_{max} \quad \textbf{[27]}$$

From [9]:

$$\begin{aligned}1-\mathbf{H} &= 1-(1-\cos\varphi)\{\mathbf{n}\}\{\mathbf{n}\}^t-\cos\varphi 1-\sin\varphi\langle\mathbf{n}\rangle \\ &= (1-\cos\varphi)1-(1-\cos\varphi)\{\mathbf{n}\}\{\mathbf{n}\}^t-\sin\varphi\langle\mathbf{n}\rangle \\ &= (1-\cos\varphi)\left[1-\{\mathbf{n}\}\{\mathbf{n}\}^t\right]-\sin\varphi\langle\mathbf{n}\rangle \\ &= (1-\cos\varphi)\langle\mathbf{n}\rangle^t\langle\mathbf{n}\rangle-\sin\varphi\langle\mathbf{n}\rangle\end{aligned} \qquad [28]$$

and from [11] and [28]:

$$\begin{aligned}\{\mathbf{n}\}^t(1-\mathbf{H}) &= \{\mathbf{n}\}^t\left[(1-\cos\varphi)\langle\mathbf{n}\rangle^t\langle\mathbf{n}\rangle-\sin\varphi\langle\mathbf{n}\rangle\right] \\ &= (1-\cos\varphi)\{\mathbf{n}\}^t\langle\mathbf{n}\rangle^t\langle\mathbf{n}\rangle-\sin\varphi\{\mathbf{n}\}^t\langle\mathbf{n}\rangle \\ &= 0\end{aligned} \qquad [29]$$

From [18] and [29]:

$$\begin{aligned}\{\mathbf{n}\}^t\{\mathbf{t}\} &= \{\mathbf{n}\}^t(1-\mathbf{H})\{\mathbf{r}_o\}+L\{\mathbf{n}\}^t\{\mathbf{n}\} \\ &= L\{\mathbf{n}\}^t\{\mathbf{n}\}=L \\ L &= \{\mathbf{n}\}^t\{\mathbf{t}\}\end{aligned} \qquad [30]$$

Thus, [30] can be used in computing L. From [18]:

$$(1-\mathbf{H})\{\mathbf{r}_o\}=\{\mathbf{t}-L\mathbf{n}\} \qquad [31]$$

Although [31] is a linear equation of $\mathbf{r}_o$, it does not yield a unique solution since any point on the helical axis will suffice [31]:

$$(1-H)\left[\{r_o\}+k\{n\}\right]=(1-H)\{r_o\}+k(1-H)\{n\}$$
$$=\{t-Ln\}+\left[(1-\cos\varphi)\langle n\rangle^t\langle n\rangle-\sin\varphi\langle n\rangle\right]\{n\}$$
$$=\{t-Ln\}$$
$$(1-H)\{r_o+kn\}=\{t-Ln\}.$$

[32]

Describe $\mathbf{r}_o$ in terms of a new vector $\mathbf{R}_o$:

$$\{r_o\}=\{R_o\}+k\{n\}$$
$$\{R_o\}^t\{n\}=0. \qquad \textbf{[33]}$$

As shown in [33], $\mathbf{R}_o$ is still the position of the helical axis but it is perpendicular to the helical axis. From [33]:

$$0=\{R_o\}^t\{n\}$$
$$=\left[\{r_o\}-k\{n\}\right]^t\{n\}=\{r_o\}^t\{n\}-k\{n\}^t\{n\}$$
$$=\{r_o\}^t\{n\}-k$$
$$k=\{r_o\}^t\{n\}$$
$$\{R_o\}=\{r_o\}-k\{n\}=\{r_o\}-\{n\}\{n\}^t\{r_o\}$$
$$=\left[1-\{n\}\{n\}^t\right]\{r_o\}$$
$$=\langle n\rangle^t\langle n\rangle\{r_o\}, \qquad \textbf{[34]}$$

and

$$\langle \mathbf{n} \rangle \{\mathbf{r}_o\} = \langle \mathbf{n} \rangle \left[\{\mathbf{R}_o\} + k\{\mathbf{n}\} \right]$$
$$= \langle \mathbf{n} \rangle \{\mathbf{R}_o\} - k\langle \mathbf{n} \rangle \{\mathbf{n}\} = \langle \mathbf{n} \rangle \{\mathbf{R}_o\}$$
$$(1 - \mathbf{H})\{\mathbf{r}_o\} = \left[(1 - \cos\varphi)\langle \mathbf{n} \rangle^t \langle \mathbf{n} \rangle - \sin\varphi \langle \mathbf{n} \rangle \right] \{\mathbf{r}_o\}$$
$$= (1 - \cos\varphi)\langle \mathbf{n} \rangle^t \langle \mathbf{n} \rangle \{\mathbf{r}_o\} - \sin\varphi \langle \mathbf{n} \rangle \{\mathbf{r}_o\}$$
$$= (1 - \cos\varphi)\{\mathbf{R}_o\} - \sin\varphi \langle \mathbf{n} \rangle \{\mathbf{R}_o\}$$
$$= \left[(1 - \cos\varphi)\mathbf{1} - \sin\varphi \langle \mathbf{n} \rangle \right] \{\mathbf{R}_o\}. \quad \textbf{[35]}$$

From [31] and [35]:

$$\left[(1 - \cos\varphi)\mathbf{1} - \sin\varphi \langle \mathbf{n} \rangle \right] \{\mathbf{R}_o\} = \{\mathbf{t} - L\mathbf{n}\}$$

$$\{\mathbf{R}_o\} = \left[(1 - \cos\varphi)\mathbf{1} - \sin\varphi \langle \mathbf{n} \rangle \right]^{-1} \cdot \{\mathbf{t} - L\mathbf{n}\}. \quad \textbf{[36]}$$

[36] has a unique solution since $\mathbf{R}_o$ is the position vector of the helical axis which is perpendicular to the helical axis.

Use [16], [19], [20], [25] or [27], [30], and [36] to obtain a complete set of description on the helical axis for a given situation.

Helical Axis vs. Transformation Matrix

[Fig. 5] shows 4 new vectors: $\mathbf{R}_i$, $\mathbf{R}_{i+1}$, $\mathbf{y}_i$, and $\mathbf{y}_{i+1}$. Vector $\mathbf{R}$ is the relative position of the origin of the reference frame fixed to the rotating body to point R while $\mathbf{y}$ is the position of a point observed in the rotating reference frame:

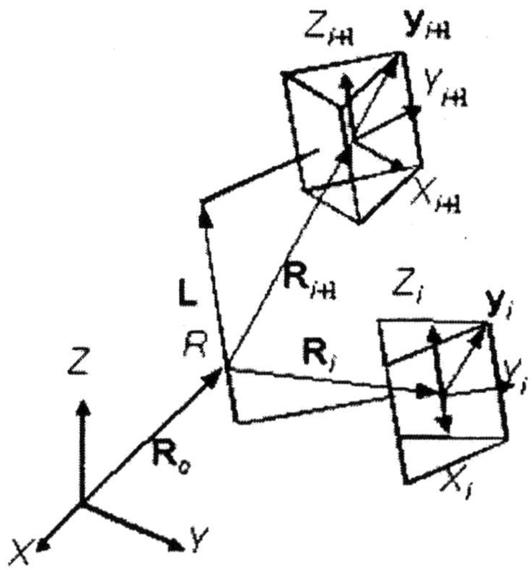

[Fig. 5]

$$\mathbf{r}_{i,j} = \mathbf{R}_o + \mathbf{R}_i + \mathbf{y}_{i,j}$$
$$\mathbf{r}_{i+1,j} = \mathbf{R}_o + \mathbf{R}_{i+1} + \mathbf{y}_{i+1,j} \quad \textbf{[37]}$$

The relative position of any point fixed to the rotating body to point R in fact suffices [14] and the origin of the local reference frame is no exception. From [14] and [Fig. 5]:

$$\{\mathbf{R}_{i+1}\} = \mathbf{H}\{\mathbf{R}_i\} + \{\mathbf{L}\}, \quad \textbf{[38]}$$

and

$$\mathbf{r}_{i+1,j} - \mathbf{R}_o = \mathbf{R}_{i+1} + \mathbf{y}_{i+1,j}$$
$$\mathbf{r}_{i,j} - \mathbf{R}_o = \mathbf{R}_i + \mathbf{y}_{i,j};$$
$$\{\mathbf{R}_{i+1} + \mathbf{y}_{i+1,j}\} = \mathbf{H}\{\mathbf{R}_i + \mathbf{y}_{i,j}\} + \{\mathbf{L}\}$$
$$\{\mathbf{R}_{i+1}\} + \{\mathbf{y}_{i+1,j}\} = \mathbf{H}\{\mathbf{R}_i\} + \mathbf{H}\{\mathbf{y}_{i,j}\} + \{\mathbf{L}\}$$
$$\{\mathbf{y}_{i+1,j}\} = \mathbf{H}\{\mathbf{y}_{i,j}\}. \quad \textbf{[39]}$$

The relative positions of the point of interest to the rotating reference frame can be transformed as

$$\{\mathbf{y}_{i,j}\} = \mathbf{T}_{i/F}{}^{t}\{\mathbf{y}_{i,j}^{(i)}\}$$
$$\{\mathbf{y}_{i+1,j}\} = \mathbf{T}_{i+1/F}{}^{t}\{\mathbf{y}_{i+1,j}^{(i+1)}\}, \quad [40]$$

where $\mathbf{T}_{i/F}$ = the transformation matrix from the fixed frame (*XYZ*-system) to frame *i* ($X_iY_iZ_i$-system), and $\mathbf{y}_i^{(i)}$ = vector $\mathbf{y}_i$ described in frame *i*, etc. From [39] and [40]:

$$\mathbf{T}_{i+1/F}{}^{t}\{\mathbf{y}_{i+1,j}^{(i+1)}\} = \mathbf{H}\cdot\mathbf{T}_{i/F}{}^{t}\{\mathbf{y}_{i,j}^{(i)}\}$$
$$\mathbf{T}_{i+1/F}{}^{t} = \mathbf{H}\cdot\mathbf{T}_{i/F}{}^{t}$$
$$\mathbf{T}_{i+1/F}{}^{t}\cdot\mathbf{T}_{i/F} = \mathbf{H} \quad [41]$$

since the local reference frame rotates with the body and the relative position of a point on the body described in its local reference frame does not change:

$$\{\mathbf{y}_{i+1,j}^{(i+1)}\} = \{\mathbf{y}_{i,j}^{(i)}\} \quad [42]$$

[41] basically shows that the helical rotation matrix can be obtained directly from the transformation matrices.

Motion Sensors: Joint Center

Rotation Matrix

Electromagnetic motion sensors typically provide with their positions and orientations at a given instant in real time. Assuming each sensor represents a rigid body, the location of the origin and the orientation of the local reference frame each sensor represents are readily available. From [41] of the Helical (Screw) Axis page:

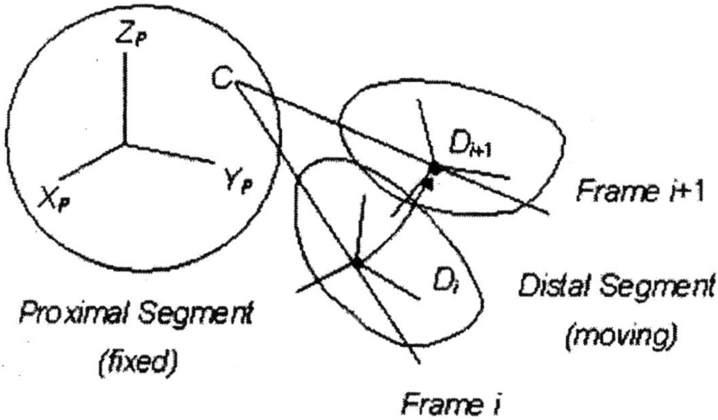

Fig. 1

$$\mathbf{R}_{D/P}^{i\to i+1} = \mathbf{T}_{D_{i+1}/P_{i+1}}{}^{t}\ \mathbf{T}_{D_i/P_i}\ , \quad \textbf{[1]}$$

where P_i = the reference frame of the linked proximal segment (fixed body) in frame i, D_i = the reference frame of the linked distal segment (moving body) in frame i, $\mathbf{R}_{D/P}^{i\to i+1}$ = the rotation matrix for the relative rotation of the distal body to the proximal body from frame i to frame i+1, and $\mathbf{T}_{A/B}$ = the rotational transformation matrix from frame B to frame A (Fig. 1). The transformation matrix from the proximal segment reference frame to the distal segment reference frame can be obtained as follows:

$$\mathbf{T}_{D_i/P_i} = \mathbf{T}_{D_i/G} \cdot \mathbf{T}_{P_i/G}{}^{t}$$
$$\mathbf{T}_{D_{i+1}/P_{i+1}} = \mathbf{T}_{D_{i+1}/G} \cdot \mathbf{T}_{P_{i+1}/G}{}^{t}\ , \quad \textbf{[2]}$$

where $\mathbf{T}_{A/G}$ = the transformation matrix from the global reference frame to frame A. The transformation matrices from the global (inertial) frame to the local (segmental) reference frames are the immediate output of the motion sensors. From [1] and [2]:

$$\mathbf{R}_{D/P}^{i\to i+1} = \left[\mathbf{T}_{D_{i+1}/G} \cdot \mathbf{T}_{P_{i+1}/G}{}^{t}\right]^{t} \cdot \mathbf{T}_{D_i/G} \cdot \mathbf{T}_{P_i/G}{}^{t}$$
$$= \mathbf{T}_{P_{i+1}/G} \cdot \mathbf{T}_{D_{i+1}/G}{}^{t} \cdot \mathbf{T}_{D_i/G} \cdot \mathbf{T}_{P_i/G}{}^{t} \qquad [3]$$

Joint Center

For a multi-DOF joint formed by two segments, proximal and distal, let vector $\mathbf{r}_{P_i}$ & $\mathbf{r}_{D_i}$ be the positions of the sensors on the proximal and distal segments (proximal and distal sensors), respectively, in frame *i*. The relative positions of the distal sensor to the proximal sensor can be described as

$$\mathbf{r}_{D/P_i} = \mathbf{r}_{D_i} - \mathbf{r}_{P_i}$$
$$\mathbf{r}_{D/P_{i+1}} = \mathbf{r}_{D_{i+1}} - \mathbf{r}_{P_{i+1}}, \qquad [4]$$

where $\mathbf{r}_{D/P_i}$ = the relative position of the distal sensor to the proximal sensor in frame *i*, etc. The relative positions observed in the proximal body reference frame become

$$\mathbf{r}_{D/P_i}^{(P_i)} = \mathbf{T}_{P_i/G} \cdot \left(\mathbf{r}_{D_i} - \mathbf{r}_{P_i}\right)$$
$$\mathbf{r}_{D/P_{i+1}}^{(P_{i+1})} = \mathbf{T}_{P_{i+1}/G} \cdot \left(\mathbf{r}_{D_{i+1}} - \mathbf{r}_{P_{i+1}}\right), \qquad [5]$$

where $\mathbf{r}^{(A)}$ = position vector described in reference frame *A*.

The relative positions of the distal sensor to the proximal sensor in frames *i* and *i*+1 suffice the following relationship:

$$\left[\mathbf{r}_{D/P_{i+1}}^{(P_{i+1})} - \mathbf{r}_c\right] = \mathbf{R}_{D/P}^{i\to i+1} \cdot \left[\mathbf{r}_{D/P_i}^{(P_i)} - \mathbf{r}_c\right]$$
$$\left(1 - \mathbf{R}_{D/P}^{i\to i+1}\right) \cdot \mathbf{r}_c = \mathbf{r}_{D/P_{i+1}}^{(P_{i+1})} - \mathbf{R}_{D/P}^{i\to i+1} \cdot \mathbf{r}_{D/P_i}^{(P_i)}$$
$$\mathbf{P}_i \cdot \mathbf{r}_c = \mathbf{Q}_i \qquad [6]$$

where $\mathbf{r}_c$ = the position of the joint center observed in the proximal reference frame, and

$$\mathbf{P}_i = \begin{bmatrix} p_{xx_i} & p_{xy_i} & p_{xz_i} \\ p_{yx_i} & p_{yy_i} & p_{yz_i} \\ p_{zx_i} & p_{zy_i} & p_{zz_i} \end{bmatrix} = \mathbf{1} - \mathbf{R}_{D/P}^{i \to i+1}$$

$$\mathbf{Q}_i = \begin{bmatrix} q_{x_i} \\ q_{y_i} \\ q_{z_i} \end{bmatrix} = \mathbf{r}_{D/P_{i+1}}^{(P_{i+1})} - \mathbf{R}_{D/P}^{i \to i+1} \cdot \mathbf{r}_{D/P_i}^{(P_i)} \quad [7]$$

In [6] it was assumed that there is no relative translation between the proximal and distal segments. [6] actually provides with 3 equations and by expanding [6] to *N* - 1 intervals a total of 3 * (*N* - 1) linear equations of $\mathbf{r}_c$ can be obtained:

$$\begin{bmatrix} p_{xx_1} & p_{xy_1} & p_{xz_1} \\ p_{yx_1} & p_{yy_1} & p_{yz_1} \\ p_{zx_1} & p_{zy_1} & p_{zz_1} \\ \cdot & \cdot & \cdot \\ p_{xx_{N-1}} & p_{xy_{N-1}} & p_{xz_{N-1}} \\ p_{yx_{N-1}} & p_{yy_{N-1}} & p_{yz_{N-1}} \\ p_{zx_{N-1}} & p_{zy_{N-1}} & p_{zz_{N-1}} \end{bmatrix} \cdot \mathbf{r}_c = \begin{bmatrix} q_{x_1} \\ q_{y_1} \\ q_{z_1} \\ \cdot \\ q_{x_{N-1}} \\ q_{y_{N-1}} \\ q_{z_{N-1}} \end{bmatrix} . \quad [8]$$

The position of the center of the multi-DOF joint observed in the proximal reference frame ($\mathbf{r}_c$) can be obtained by solving [8] through the least square approach.

Once $\mathbf{r}_c$ is known, the global position of the joint center in each frame can be computed:

$$\mathbf{R}_{ci} = \mathbf{r}_{Ai} + \mathbf{T}_{A/G}{}^{t} \cdot \mathbf{r}_c, \quad [9]$$

where $\mathbf{R}_{ci}$ = the global position of the joint center in frame *i*.

Orientation Angles -- Eulerian/Cardanian Angles

Since the rotation matrices, [2], [3] & [4] of Rotation Matrix are transformation matrices, one can perform successive rotations to transform a vector from one reference frame to another.

The sequence of the successive rotations can vary depending on the intention of the analyst. There are two typical types of successive rotations: **Eulerian** and **Cardanian**. The Eulerian type involves repetition of rotations about one particular axis:

XYX, *XZX*, *YXY*, *YZY*, *ZXZ*, *ZYZ*. The Cardanian type is characterized by the rotations about all three axes: *XYZ*, *XZY*, *YZX*, *YXZ*, *ZXY*, *ZYX*. The sequence of the successive rotations can be chosen from a total of 12 different combinations. Even though the Cardanian type is different from the Eulerian type in terms of the combination of the rotations, they both use very similar approach to compute the orientation angles.

One may treat the Cardanian sequences as a subset of the Eulerian. For simplicity, only the *XYZ*-type successive rotations (Figure 1) will be explored here.

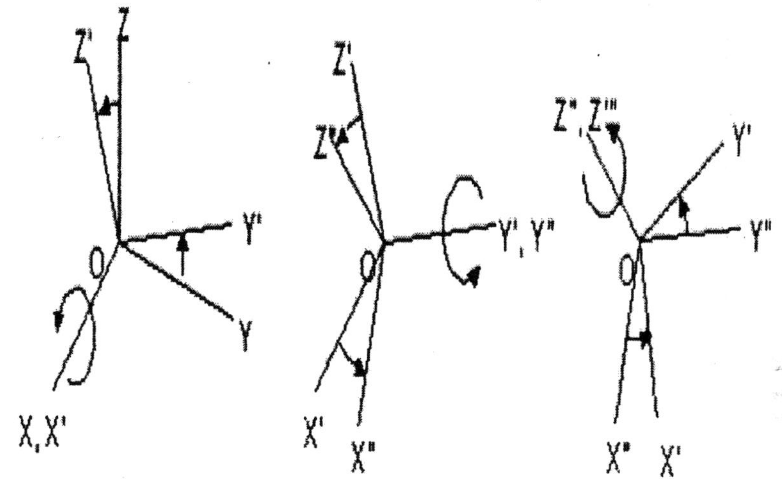

Figure 1

Figure 1 shows three successive rotations to change the orientation of the reference frame from the *XYZ* system to the *X'''Y'''Z'''* system. The intermediate systems are denoted as *X'Y'Z'* system and *X''Y''Z''* system, respectively:

$$\begin{bmatrix} x' \\ y' \\ z' \end{bmatrix} = \begin{bmatrix} 1 & 0 & 0 \\ 0 & c(\phi) & s(\phi) \\ 0 & -s(\phi) & c(\phi) \end{bmatrix} \cdot \begin{bmatrix} x \\ y \\ z \end{bmatrix}$$

$$\begin{bmatrix} x'' \\ y'' \\ z'' \end{bmatrix} = \begin{bmatrix} c(\theta) & 0 & -s(\theta) \\ 0 & 1 & 0 \\ s(\theta) & 0 & c(\theta) \end{bmatrix} \cdot \begin{bmatrix} x' \\ y' \\ z' \end{bmatrix}$$

$$\begin{bmatrix} x''' \\ y''' \\ z''' \end{bmatrix} = \begin{bmatrix} c(\psi) & s(\psi) & 0 \\ -s(\psi) & c(\psi) & 0 \\ 0 & 0 & 1 \end{bmatrix} \cdot \begin{bmatrix} x'' \\ y'' \\ z'' \end{bmatrix} \quad [1]$$

where, *c*( ) = cos, and *s*( ) = sin. The successive rotations can be expressed as multiplication of the rotation matrices

The axis of the second rotation (rotation by angle *q*) is the *Y* axis of the intermediate frames, *Y'* / *Y"* axis in Figure 1, not that of either frame *A* or frame *B*. This sometimes causes confusion in assigning practical meanings to the orientation angles. In our example above (pelvis vs. right thigh), the thigh adduction/abduction occurs not in the frontal plane of the pelvis, but in the intermediate frontal plane of the right thigh. In other words, angle θ in this example is not the same to the anatomical adduction/abduction angle. The anatomical joint-motion angles are actually the projected angles, not the orientation angles.

The orientation angles are sequence-dependent so that you will get different sets of orientation angles from different sequences of successive rotations. In other word, type *YXZ* provides orientation angle values different from those of type *XYZ*. It is up to the analyst to choose the type of successive rotations, but employing different rotation sequences for different segments will complicate the analysis quite a bit.

Computation of the Orientation Angles

One can compute the transformation matrices based on the global coordinates of the markers. Let

$$\mathbf{T} \equiv \begin{bmatrix} t_{11} & t_{12} & t_{13} \\ t_{21} & t_{22} & t_{23} \\ t_{31} & t_{32} & t_{33} \end{bmatrix} \quad [4]$$

From [3] and [4]:

$$\begin{bmatrix} t_{11} & t_{12} & t_{13} \\ t_{21} & t_{22} & t_{23} \\ t_{31} & t_{32} & t_{33} \end{bmatrix} = \begin{bmatrix} c(\theta)c(\psi) & s(\phi)s(\theta)c(\psi)+c(\phi)s(\psi) & -c(\phi)s(\theta)c(\psi)+s(\phi)s(\psi) \\ -c(\theta)s(\psi) & -s(\phi)s(\theta)s(\psi)+c(\phi)c(\psi) & c(\phi)s(\theta)s(\psi)+s(\phi)c(\psi) \\ s(\theta) & -s(\phi)c(\theta) & c(\phi)c(\theta) \end{bmatrix} \quad [5]$$

Therefore:

$$\theta = \begin{cases} \sin^{-1}(t_{31}) \\ \quad or \\ \pi - \sin^{-1}(t_{31}) \end{cases} \quad [6]$$

and

if $\theta \neq \pm\frac{\pi}{2}$:

$$\phi = \begin{cases} \tan^{-1}\left[\frac{-t_{32}}{t_{33}}\right] & (t_{33} \cdot \cos\ \theta > 0) \\ \tan^{-1}\left[\frac{-t_{32}}{t_{33}}\right] + \pi & (t_{33} \cdot \cos\ \theta < 0) \end{cases}$$

$$\psi = \begin{cases} \tan^{-1}\left[\frac{-t_{21}}{t_{11}}\right] & (t_{11} \cdot \cos\ \theta > 0) \\ \tan^{-1}\left[\frac{-t_{21}}{t_{11}}\right] + \pi & (t_{11} \cos\ \theta < 0) \end{cases}$$

[7a & b]

From [6] & [7], one can obtain two different sets of orientation angles but must pay attention to the time history of the second orientation angle (θ) to choose the right set of orientation angles. In many cases one may assume $-\pi/2 < \theta < \pi/2$. For example, the inclination angle shown in Figure 2 can not be larger than $\pi/2$ rad or smaller than $-\pi/2$ rad and one will get only one set of orientation angles as a result. But this may not be true in the case of the relative orientation angles of a segment to its proximal segment at a ball-and-socket joint. In shoulder abduction, for example, the abduction angle continuously increases and gets larger than $\pi/2$ rad or smaller than $-\pi/2$ rad. One must exercise caution in dealing with θ in different situations.

Now, let's take a look at a special case. From [4] & [5]:

$$\text{if } \theta = \pm\frac{\pi}{2}:$$

$$\sin\theta = \pm 1, \ \cos\theta = 0$$

$$\begin{bmatrix} c(\theta)c(\psi) & s(\phi)s(\theta)c(\psi)+c(\phi)s(\psi) & -c(\phi)s(\theta)c(\psi)+s(\phi)s(\psi) \\ -c(\theta)s(\psi) & -s(\phi)s(\theta)s(\psi)+c(\phi)c(\psi) & c(\phi)s(\theta)s(\psi)+s(\phi)c(\psi) \\ s(\theta) & -s(\phi)c(\theta) & c(\phi)c(\theta) \end{bmatrix}$$

$$= \begin{bmatrix} 0 & \pm s(\phi)c(\psi)+c(\phi)s(\psi) & \mp c(\phi)c(\psi)+s(\phi)s(\psi) \\ 0 & \mp s(\phi)s(\psi)+c(\phi)c(\psi) & \pm c(\phi)s(\psi)+s(\phi)c(\psi) \\ \pm 1 & 0 & 0 \end{bmatrix}$$

$$= \begin{bmatrix} 0 & \pm[s(\phi)c(\psi)\pm c(\phi)s(\psi)] & \mp[c(\phi)c(\psi)\mp s(\phi)s(\psi)] \\ 0 & c(\phi)c(\psi)\mp s(\phi)s(\psi) & s(\phi)c(\psi)\pm c(\phi)s(\psi) \\ \pm 1 & 0 & 0 \end{bmatrix}$$

$$= \begin{bmatrix} 0 & \pm s(\phi\pm\psi) & \mp c(\phi\pm\psi) \\ 0 & c(\phi\pm\psi) & s(\phi\pm\psi) \\ \pm 1 & 0 & 0 \end{bmatrix}$$

[8]

Therefore:

$$\phi \pm \psi = \begin{cases} \tan^{-1}\left[\dfrac{t_{23}}{t_{22}}\right] & (t_{22} > 0) \\ \tan^{-1}\left[\dfrac{-t_{23}}{t_{22}}\right] + \pi & (t_{22} < 0) \end{cases}$$

[9]

In other words, if cos θ = 0, one can not compute ϕ and ψ separately, but collectively as $\phi + \psi$ or $\phi - \psi$. These conditions are called the **gimbal locks**.

One can compute the angular velocity of a rigid body using the orientation angles. See Angular Velocity vs Orientation Angles for the details.

Relative Transformation at the Joint

The main task in the joint kinematics is to compute the relative orientation angles of the segments to their respective proximally-linked segments at the joints. This is done based on the local reference frames of the segments defined. The segmental reference frames can be obtained from the coordinates of the markers and joint centers. For example, the unit coordinate vectors of the pelvis and the right thigh shown in Figure 1 can be obtained as follows:

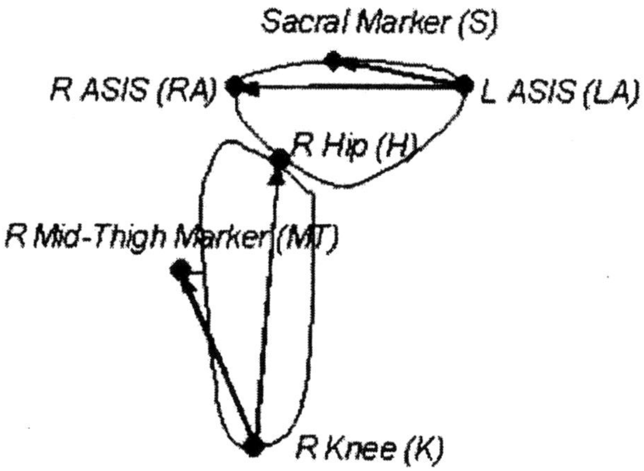

Figure 1

$$\mathbf{i}_{PL} = \frac{\mathbf{r}_{RA} - \mathbf{r}_{LA}}{|\mathbf{r}_{RA} - \mathbf{r}_{LA}|}$$

$$\mathbf{k}_{PL} = \frac{(\mathbf{r}_S - \mathbf{r}_{LA}) \times \mathbf{i}_{PL}}{|(\mathbf{r}_S - \mathbf{r}_{LA}) \times \mathbf{i}_{PL}|}$$

$$\mathbf{j}_{PL} = \mathbf{k}_{PL} \times \mathbf{i}_{PL} \quad , \quad [1]$$

and

$$\mathbf{k}_{TH} = \frac{\mathbf{r}_H - \mathbf{r}_K}{|\mathbf{r}_H - \mathbf{r}_K|}$$

$$\mathbf{j}_{TH} = \frac{\mathbf{k}_{TH} \times (\mathbf{r}_{MT} - \mathbf{r}_K)}{|\mathbf{k}_{TH} \times (\mathbf{r}_{MT} - \mathbf{r}_K)|}$$

$$\mathbf{i}_{TH} = \mathbf{j}_{TH} \times \mathbf{k}_{TH} \quad , \quad [2]$$

where **i**, **j** & **k** = the unit coordinate vectors. Describing the unit coordinate vectors as row matrices:

$$\mathbf{i} \equiv \begin{bmatrix} t_{11} & t_{12} & t_{13} \end{bmatrix}$$

$$\mathbf{j} \equiv \begin{bmatrix} t_{21} & t_{22} & t_{23} \end{bmatrix}$$

$$\mathbf{k} \equiv \begin{bmatrix} t_{31} & t_{32} & t_{33} \end{bmatrix} . \quad [3]$$

See Transformation Matrix in the Axis Transformation section for the details. The unit coordinate vectors of the segmental reference frames form the transformation matrices from the global frame, respectively:

$$\mathbf{T}_{P/G} = \begin{bmatrix} \mathbf{i}_P \\ \mathbf{j}_P \\ \mathbf{k}_P \end{bmatrix} = \begin{bmatrix} t_{11P} & t_{12P} & t_{13P} \\ t_{21P} & t_{22P} & t_{23P} \\ t_{31P} & t_{32P} & t_{33P} \end{bmatrix}$$

$$\mathbf{T}_{D/G} = \begin{bmatrix} \mathbf{i}_D \\ \mathbf{j}_D \\ \mathbf{k}_D \end{bmatrix} = \begin{bmatrix} t_{11D} & t_{12D} & t_{13D} \\ t_{21D} & t_{22D} & t_{23D} \\ t_{31D} & t_{32D} & t_{33D} \end{bmatrix} , \quad [4]$$

where P = the proximal segment, D = the distal segment, and G = the global inertial reference frame. The transformation matrix from the proximal reference frame (frame P) to the distal reference frame

D) can be computed from the transformation matrices shown

$$\mathbf{T}_{D/P} = \mathbf{T}_{D/G}\mathbf{T}_{G/P} = \mathbf{T}_{D/G}\mathbf{T}_{P/G}{}^{t} = \begin{bmatrix} t_{11J} & t_{12J} & t_{13J} \\ t_{21J} & t_{22J} & t_{23J} \\ t_{31J} & t_{32J} & t_{33J} \end{bmatrix} \quad , \quad [5]$$

where *J* stands for the joint involved. See the Transformation Matrix page for the details of computation of the transformation matrix from one local frame to another.

From [5] of Orientation Angles in the Axis Transformation section:

$$\begin{bmatrix} t_{11J} & t_{12J} & t_{13J} \\ t_{21J} & t_{22J} & t_{23J} \\ t_{31J} & t_{32J} & t_{33J} \end{bmatrix} = \begin{bmatrix} c(\theta_J)c(\psi_J) & s(\phi_J)s(\theta_J)c(\psi_J)+c(\phi_J)s(\psi_J) & -c(\phi_J)s(\theta_J)c(\psi_J)+s(\phi_J)s(\psi_J) \\ -c(\theta_J)s(\psi_J) & -s(\phi_J)s(\theta_J)s(\psi_J)+c(\phi_J)c(\psi_J) & c(\phi_J)s(\theta_J)s(\psi_J)+s(\phi_J)c(\psi_J) \\ s(\theta_J) & -s(\phi_J)c(\theta_J) & c(\phi_J)c(\theta_J) \end{bmatrix} \quad , \quad [6]$$

where ϕ, θ & ψ = the relative orientation angles of the distal segment to the proximal segment forming the joint, $c(x) = \cos x$, and $s(x) = \sin x$.

Computation of θ_J

In [7], θ_J is the first angle to compute. The general solutions of angle θ_J are

$$\theta_J = \begin{cases} 1) & \sin^{-1}(t_{31J}) + 2\pi n \\ 2) & \pm\pi - \sin^{-1}(t_{31J}) + 2\pi n \end{cases} \quad (n = \ldots -2, -1, 0, 1, 2, \ldots) \quad , \quad [7]$$

where n = integer number which is quite likely to be 0 for angle θ_J. As shown in [7], two possible solutions can be obtained as θ_J. The return value of the inverse sine function ($\sin^{-1}$) ranges

$$-\frac{\pi}{2} \le \sin^{-1}(x) \le \frac{\pi}{2} \qquad [8]$$

Since angle θ is the orientation angle about the Y axis, it generally stays within the range shown in [8] with one exception: the shoulder. In the shoulder, angle θ_J can be outside the range shown in [8]. Let's use the shoulder abduction from the anatomical reference frame as an example. The abduction angle in fact coincides with angle θ_J in this case and the abduction angle can obviously exceed $\pi/2$ (90°) as shown in Figure 2. The red arrow in the figure shows the motion of the upperarm from position 1 to position 2, passing the 90° position.

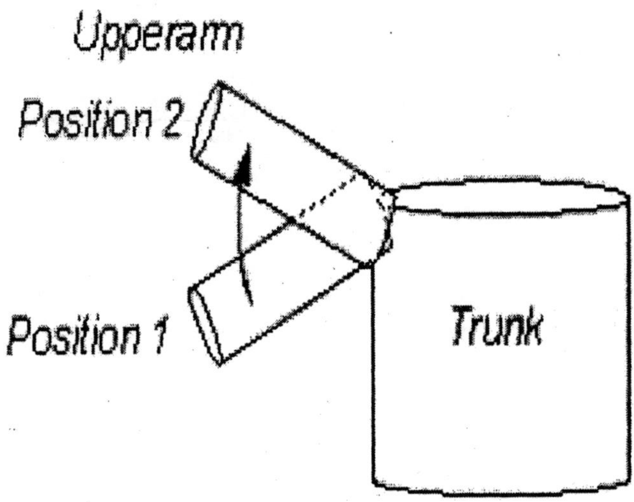

Figure 2

The more direct and useful solutions for angle θ_J would be

$$\theta_J = \begin{cases} 1) & \sin^{-1}(t_{31J}) \\ 2) & \dfrac{t_{31J}}{|t_{31J}|}\pi - \sin^{-1}(t_{31J}) \end{cases} \quad [9]$$

The solutions shown in [9] are in the range of

$$-\pi \leq \theta_J < \pi \quad [10]$$

In Figure 3, the purple arrows represent case 1 shown in [9]. In order to bring the upperarm reference frame to position 2 in this case, one must first flex the shoulder (ϕ_J) by π. Therefore, one will observe discontinuity in ϕ_J between positions 1 and 2 while θ_J remains smaller than $\pi/2$. On the other hand, the blue arrow represents case 2 shown in [9]. Angle ϕ_J stays (= 0) while angle θ_J passes and becomes larger than $\pi/2$. One can only find the true solution by considering the continuous motion of the upperarm.

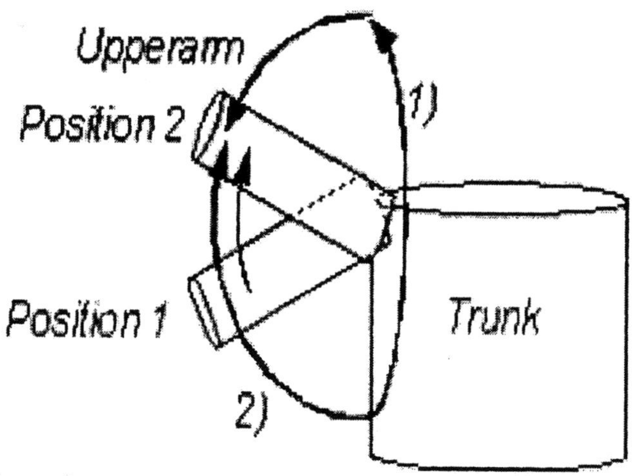

Figure 3

Computation of ϕ_J and ψ_J

Once θ_J is known, ϕ_J and ψ_J can be computed. In both cases, the sine and cosine of the angle are given and one can use the inverse tangent ($\tan^{-1}$) function for this job. The general solution are

$\sin\theta_J \neq \pm 1$:

$$\phi_J = \begin{cases} \tan^{-1}\left(\dfrac{-t_{32J}}{t_{33J}}\right) + 2\pi n & (t_{33J}\cos\theta_J > 0) \\ \tan^{-1}\left(\dfrac{-t_{32J}}{t_{33J}}\right) \pm \pi + 2\pi n & (t_{33J}\cos\theta_J < 0) \end{cases} \quad (n = \ldots, -2, -1, 0, 1, 2, \ldots)$$

$$\psi_J = \begin{cases} \tan^{-1}\left(\dfrac{-t_{21J}}{t_{11J}}\right) + 2\pi n & (t_{11J}\cos\theta_J > 0) \\ +2\pi n & (t_{11J}\cos\theta_J < 0) \end{cases} \quad (n = \ldots, -2, -1, 0, 1, 2, \ldots)$$

where n = integer number which is not necessarily 0, especially in the shoulder joint. In addition, n may not be zero when one computes the relative orientation of a particular segment to the global frame if the motion involves multiple somersaults and/or twists. n must be figured out considering the continuity in the angle.

Although the return value of the inverse tangent function ranges

$$-\frac{\pi}{2} < \tan^{-1}(x) < \frac{\pi}{2}, \quad [12]$$

one can compute the true angle since both the sine and cosine of the angle are given. The angle range shown in [12] coincides with that of positive cosine. The more specific solution would be

$$\phi_J = \begin{cases} \tan^{-1}\left(\dfrac{-t_{32J}}{t_{33J}}\right) + 2\pi n & (t_{33J}\cos\theta_J > 0) \\ \tan^{-1}\left(\dfrac{-t_{32J}}{t_{33J}}\right) + \pi + 2\pi n & (t_{33J}\cos\theta_J < 0,\ t_{32J}\cos\theta_J < 0) \\ \tan^{-1}\left(\dfrac{-t_{32J}}{t_{33J}}\right) - \pi + 2\pi n & (t_{33J}\cos\theta_J < 0,\ t_{32J}\cos\theta_J \geq 0) \\ \dfrac{\pi}{2} + 2\pi n & (t_{33J}\cos\theta_J = 0,\ t_{32J}\cos\theta_J < 0) \\ -\dfrac{\pi}{2} + 2\pi n & (t_{33J}\cos\theta_J = 0,\ t_{32J}\cos\theta_J > 0) \end{cases}$$

, **[13]**

and

$$\psi_J = \begin{cases} \tan^{-1}\left(\dfrac{-t_{21J}}{t_{11J}}\right) + 2\pi n & (t_{11J}\cos\theta_J > 0) \\ \tan^{-1}\left(\dfrac{-t_{21J}}{t_{11J}}\right) + \pi + 2\pi n & (t_{11J}\cos\theta_J < 0,\ t_{21J}\cos\theta_J < 0) \\ \tan^{-1}\left(\dfrac{-t_{21J}}{t_{11J}}\right) - \pi + 2\pi n & (t_{11J}\cos\theta_J < 0,\ t_{21J}\cos\theta_J \geq 0) \\ \dfrac{\pi}{2} + 2\pi n & (t_{11J}\cos\theta_J = 0,\ t_{21J}\cos\theta_J < 0) \\ -\dfrac{\pi}{2} + 2\pi n & (t_{11J}\cos\theta_J = 0,\ t_{21J}\cos\theta_J > 0) \end{cases}$$

[14]

In [13] and [14]:

$$t_{33J}\cos\theta_J = (\cos\phi_J \cos\theta_J)\cos\theta_J = \cos\phi_J \cos^2\theta_J$$
$$t_{32J}\cos\theta_J = (-\cos\theta_J \sin\psi_J)\cos\theta_J = -\cos^2\theta_J \sin\psi_J$$
$$\vdots$$
$$t_{33J}\cos\theta_J > 0 \Leftrightarrow \cos\phi_J > 0$$
$$t_{32J}\cos\theta_J > 0 \Leftrightarrow \sin\phi_J < 0$$
$$t_{11J}\cos\theta_J > 0 \Leftrightarrow \cos\psi_J > 0$$
$$t_{21J}\cos\theta_J > 0 \Leftrightarrow \sin\psi_J < 0$$
$$\vdots \qquad [15]$$

In the case of the gimbal lock, [6] reduces to

$$\sin\theta_J = \pm 1:$$
$$\begin{bmatrix} t_{11J} & t_{12J} & t_{13J} \\ t_{21J} & t_{22J} & t_{23J} \\ t_{31J} & t_{32J} & t_{33J} \end{bmatrix} = \begin{bmatrix} 0 & \pm s(\phi_J \pm \psi_J) & \mp c(\phi_J \pm \psi_J) \\ 0 & c(\phi_J \pm \psi_J) & s(\phi_J \pm \psi_J) \\ \pm 1 & 0 & 0 \end{bmatrix} \qquad [16]$$

[13] & [14] can be then modified to

$$\phi_J + t_{31J}\psi_J = \begin{cases} \tan^{-1}\left(\dfrac{t_{23J}}{t_{22J}}\right) + 2\pi n & (t_{22J} > 0) \\ \tan^{-1}\left(\dfrac{t_{23J}}{t_{22J}}\right) + \pi + 2\pi n & (t_{22J} < 0,\ t_{23J} > 0) \\ \tan^{-1}\left(\dfrac{t_{23J}}{t_{22J}}\right) - \pi + 2\pi n & (t_{22J} < 0,\ t_{23J} \le 0) \\ \dfrac{\pi}{2} + 2\pi n & (t_{22J} = 0,\ t_{23J} > 0) \\ -\dfrac{\pi}{2} + 2\pi n & (t_{22J} = 0,\ t_{23J} < 0) \end{cases} \qquad [17]$$

Again, [13], [14] & [17] provide the orientation angles in the range of

$$-\pi \leq \phi_J, \psi_J < \pi \quad [18]$$

Continuous Angles

There are two obstacles in computing the orientation angles of the distal reference frame to the proximal reference frame. Firstly, [9], [13], [14] & [17] provide two sets of orientation angles due to two possible θ_J's.

Secondly, the arbitrary integer n in [13], [14] & [17] needs to be determined. But these obstacles have a common root: continuity in the angles. In other words, the true solution and n must be determined based on the continuous relative motion of the distal reference frame to the proximal frame.

Determination of n can be taken care using the procedure explained in the Continuous Angle page in the User-Angle Issues section.

Therefore the only real problem is to choose the true orientation angle set from the two sets computed. The key to solution for this problem is the fact that one must observe discontinuity in ϕ_J and ψ_J if wrong θ_J is chosen. Thus, the angle set that shows smaller

$$|\Delta\phi_J| + |\Delta\psi_J| \quad [19]$$

Although joint angle is commonly computed from the coordinates of the joint centers as a user-angle (see the User-Angle Issues section for the details), it can be also computed from the relative orientation angles of the joint.

In 1-DOF joints such as the hinge joint, the joint angle corresponds to one of the orientation angles and no additional computation is required. But in joints with more than 1 DOF, additional computation must be performed to obtain the joint angle.

From [6] of Computation of the Orientation Angles:

rigid bodies. Among these, the simplest mechanical system that can move is a particle. A particle has mass but no volume: **mass point**. Particles are the building blocks of a rigid body. The equations for a particle will be later used to develop those for a system of particles and a rigid body. Some of the important mechanical quantities of a particle are classified and summarized on the following pages:

- Kinematics
- Linear Kinetics
- Angular Kinetics

Kinematics is basically 'the study of description of motion'. while **kinetics** is 'the study of explanation of motion'. **Description** focuses on the effects (motion) while **explanation** focuses on the cause (force & torque). Explanation requires the info about the object in motion. When one tries to explain someone else's behavior, one must know that person's personality. The personality of the object in motion is its **inertial properties** such as the mass and the moment of inertia. It is safe to say that any mechanical quantity that involves mass or moment of inertia in its equation is a kinetic quantity, such as force, momentum, energy, etc. Since the inertial properties are known, one can relate the cause (force & torque) and effects (motion) in the kinetics. On the other hand, kinematic quantities have no reference to the inertial properties of the object at all, such as in position, velocity and acceleration.

Kinematics

Position

Position of a particle is its location at a given instance. In order to specifically describe the position of a particle, we need a frame of reference or a **reference frame**. Depending on the situation, one may use a **Cartesian coordinate system** or a **polar coordinate system** to describe the position.

Position vector is the vector drawn from the origin of the reference frame to the particle's location. In Figure 1, the position of particle *P* becomes

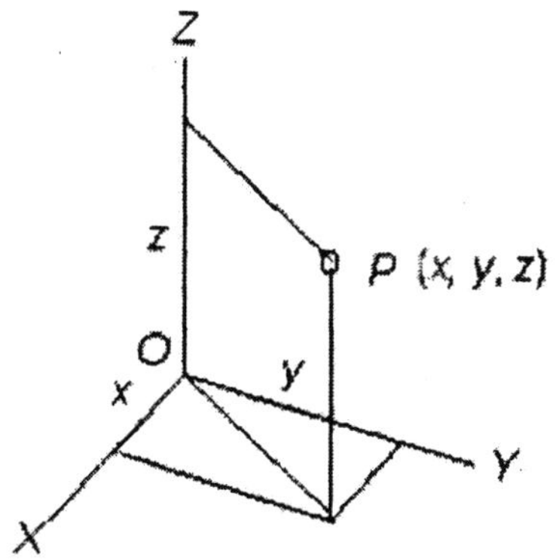

Figure 1

$$\mathbf{r} = \mathbf{i}x + \mathbf{j}y + \mathbf{k}z$$
$$= (x, y, z) \qquad [1]$$

where **i**, **j** & **k** = the unit vectors, and x, y & z = the Cartesian coordinates. One may also use a polar coordinate system (Figure 2) to describe the position:

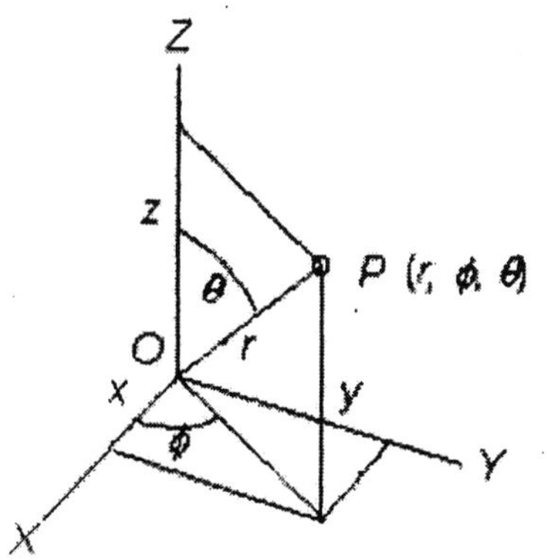

Figure 2

$$\mathbf{r} = (r, \phi, \theta) \qquad [2]$$

From [1] & [2]:

$$r=\sqrt{x^2+y^2+z^2}$$

$$\phi=\begin{cases}\tan^{-1}\left(\dfrac{y}{x}\right) & (x>0)\\ \tan^{-1}\left(\dfrac{y}{x}\right)+\pi & (x<0,y>0)\\ \tan^{-1}\left(\dfrac{y}{x}\right)-\pi & (x<0,y<0)\\ \dfrac{\pi}{2} & (x=0,y>0)\\ -\dfrac{\pi}{2} & (x=0,y<0)\end{cases}$$

$$\theta=\begin{cases}\tan^{-1}\left(\dfrac{\sqrt{x^2+y^2}}{z}\right) & (z>0)\\ \tan^{-1}\left(\dfrac{\sqrt{x^2+y^2}}{z}\right)+\pi & (z<0)\\ \dfrac{\pi}{2} & (z=0)\end{cases} \quad [3]$$

and

$$x=(r\cdot\sin\theta)\cdot\cos\phi=r\cdot\cos\phi\cdot\sin\theta$$
$$y=(r\cdot\sin\theta)\cdot\sin\phi=r\cdot\sin\phi\cdot\sin\theta$$
$$z=r\cdot\cos\theta \quad [4]$$

Velocity

Velocity is defined as the rate of change in position or the rate of displacement. From Figure 3:

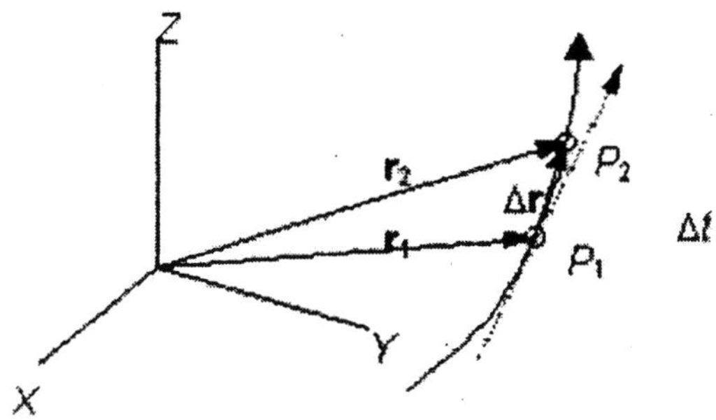

Figure 3

$$\mathbf{v} = \lim_{\Delta t \to 0} \frac{\Delta \mathbf{r}}{\Delta t} = \frac{d\mathbf{r}}{dt} \quad [5]$$

or

$$\begin{aligned} \mathbf{v} &= \frac{d\mathbf{r}}{dt} \\ &= \mathbf{i}\frac{dx}{dt} + \mathbf{j}\frac{dy}{dt} + \mathbf{k}\frac{dz}{dt} \\ &= \mathbf{i}\dot{x} + \mathbf{j}\dot{y} + \mathbf{k}\dot{z} \\ &= [\dot{x}, \dot{y}, \dot{z}] \end{aligned} \quad [6]$$

One can obtain the velocity components by taking time-derivatives of the coordinates as shown in [6]. The direction of the instantaneous velocity is along the line passing P_1 and tangential to the trajectory (dotted line) in Figure 3.

Acceleration

Acceleration is defined as the rate of change in velocity or:

$$\mathbf{a} = \lim_{\Delta t \to 0} \frac{\Delta \mathbf{v}}{\Delta t} = \frac{d\mathbf{v}}{dt}$$
$$= \mathbf{i}\frac{d\dot{x}}{dt} + \mathbf{j}\frac{d\dot{y}}{dt} + \mathbf{k}\frac{d\dot{z}}{dt} = \mathbf{i}\ddot{x} + \mathbf{j}\ddot{y} + \mathbf{k}\ddot{z} = [\ddot{x}, \ddot{y}, \ddot{z}]$$
$$= \frac{d^2\mathbf{r}}{dt^2} \quad [7]$$

From [5] and [7], it is clear that velocity is the first time-derivative of position, and acceleration is the second time-derivative of position. The first product of the motion analysis is the positions of the markers. Therefore, one can compute the velocities and accelerations of the markers through time-derivation of the position data.

Linear Kinetics

Force

Force acting on a particle is equal to the product of its mass and acceleration:

$$\mathbf{F} = m\mathbf{a} \quad [1]$$

From [1]:

$$\mathbf{a} = \frac{\mathbf{F}}{m} \quad [2]$$

The acceleration of a particle is proportional to the force acting on it and is inversely proportional to its mass: Newton's second law of motion - law of acceleration. When the force acting on a particle is zero, the acceleration is also zero: Newton's first law of motion - law of inertia.

For every action of force, there is an equal and opposite reaction: Newton's third law of motion - law of reaction. Newton's third law basically reflects the bilateral nature of the force exertion.

Momentum

Momentum of a particle is defined as the amount of motion the particle possesses which is in fact equal to the product of its mass and velocity:

$$\mathbf{p} = m\mathbf{v} \quad [3]$$

From [1]:

$$\mathbf{F} = \frac{d\mathbf{p}}{dt} \quad [4]$$

since

$$\begin{aligned}\frac{d\mathbf{p}}{dt} &= \frac{d}{dt}(m\mathbf{v}) \\ &= m\frac{d\mathbf{v}}{dt} \\ &= m\mathbf{a} \\ &= \mathbf{F} \quad [5]\end{aligned}$$

Or

$$\mathbf{p} = \int_{t_o}^{t} \mathbf{F}\ dt + \mathbf{p}_o \quad [6]$$

where $\mathbf{p}_o$ = the initial momentum of the particle, t = time, and t_o = the initial time. From [6]:

$$\begin{aligned}\Delta\mathbf{p} &= \mathbf{p} - \mathbf{p}_o \\ &= \int_{t_o}^{t} \mathbf{F} \cdot dt = \mathbf{I} \quad [7]\end{aligned}$$

where **I** = the impulse, the accumulated effect of force exertion on the particle. In other words, the impulse is equal to the change in momentum. Force exertion on the particle causes change in momentum.

Kinetic Energy

The kinetic energy of a particle is the energy due to the motion of the particle:

$$\begin{aligned} T &= \frac{1}{2}mv^2 = \frac{1}{2}m\mathbf{v}\bullet\mathbf{v} \\ &= \frac{1}{2}\mathbf{v}\bullet(m\mathbf{v}) \\ &= \frac{1}{2}\mathbf{v}\bullet\mathbf{p} \end{aligned} \quad [8]$$

Angular Kinetics

Torque

The torque or the rotating force acting on a particle with respect to the origin of the reference frame is defined as

$$\mathbf{M} = \mathbf{r} \times \mathbf{F} \quad [1]$$

where **r** = the position vector of the particle, and **F** = the force acting on the particle. [1] can be rewritten as

$$\begin{aligned} \mathbf{M} &= \mathbf{r} \times \mathbf{F} \\ &= \mathbf{r} \times \frac{d\mathbf{p}}{dt} \\ &= \frac{d}{dt}(\mathbf{r} \times \mathbf{p}) \end{aligned} \quad [2]$$

since

$$\frac{d}{dt}(\mathbf{r}\times\mathbf{p})=\frac{d\mathbf{r}}{dt}\times\mathbf{p}+\mathbf{r}\times\frac{d\mathbf{p}}{dt}$$
$$=\mathbf{v}\times\mathbf{p}+\mathbf{r}\times\frac{d\mathbf{p}}{dt}$$
$$=\mathbf{v}\times(m\mathbf{v})+\mathbf{r}\times\frac{d\mathbf{p}}{dt}$$
$$=\mathbf{r}\times\frac{d\mathbf{p}}{dt} \quad [3]$$

Angular Momentum

[2] can be rewritten as

$$\mathbf{M}=\frac{d\mathbf{H}}{dt} \quad [4]$$

where

$$\mathbf{H}=\mathbf{r}\times\mathbf{p} \quad [5]$$

H shown in [4] & [5] is the angular momentum of the particle. Angular momentum is defined as the amount of the angular motion.

From [4]:

$$\mathbf{H}=\int_{t_0}^{t}\mathbf{M}\cdot dt+\mathbf{H}_0 \quad [6]$$

where t = the time, t_0 = the initial time, and $\mathbf{H}_0$ = the initial angular momentum at t_0. From [6], the angular impulse is the accumulated effect of the torque exertion on the particle:

$$\Delta\mathbf{H}=\mathbf{H}-\mathbf{H}_0$$
$$=\int_{t_0}^{t}\mathbf{M}\ dt \quad [7]$$

Dynamics of a System Particles

A system of particles means a group of particles inter-related. The equations for a system of particles can be readily used to develop those for a rigid body. One new but very important concept introduced with a system of particles is the **center of mass**. The following quantities are covered in this section:

- Center of Mass (CM)
- Momentum
- Angular Momentum

Kinetic Energy

The equations for linear motion variables such as CM and momentum are generally very simple. But those for the angular motion variables become bit more complex than those for a particle. These equations will be further developed in the Rigid Body Dynamics section.

First Mass Moment

The **1st mass moment** of a particle is defined as the product of its mass and position vector (Figure 1):

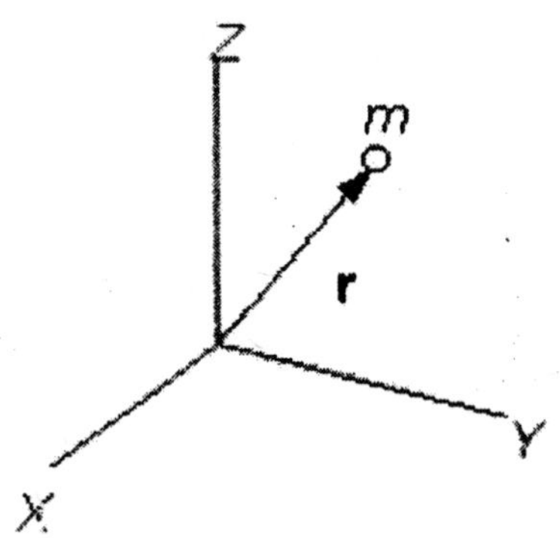

Figure 1

$$\mathbf{q} = m\mathbf{r} \quad [1]$$

where **q** = the first mass moment, m = the mass, and **r** = the position vector. The total mass moment of the system of particles shown in Figure 2 is then

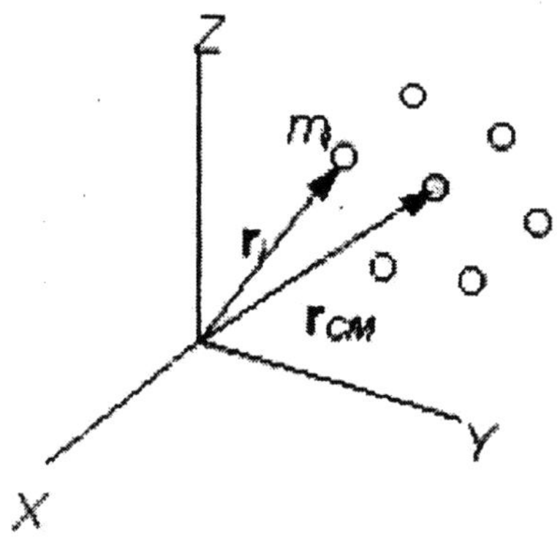

Figure 2

$$\mathbf{q} = \sum_i \mathbf{q}_i = \sum_i m_i \mathbf{r}_i \qquad [2]$$

where i = point number.

Center of Mass

Center of mass is an imaginary point which suffices the following relationship:

$$\mathbf{q} = \sum_i m_i \mathbf{r}_i = \left(\sum_i m_i\right) \cdot \mathbf{r}_{CM} = m_{total} \mathbf{r}_{CM} \qquad [3]$$

where m_{total} = the mass of the system, $\mathbf{r}_{CM}$ = the position vector of the CM. In other words, the CM is a single point which effectively represents the whole system. From [3]:

$$\mathbf{r}_{CM} = \frac{\mathbf{q}}{m_{total}} = \frac{\sum_i m_i \mathbf{r}_i}{\sum_i m_i}$$

$$= \left[\frac{\sum_i m_i x_i}{\sum_i m_i}, \frac{\sum_i m_i y_i}{\sum_i m_i}, \frac{\sum_i m_i z_i}{\sum_i m_i} \right] \quad [4]$$

Based on Figure 3, [2] can be rewritten as

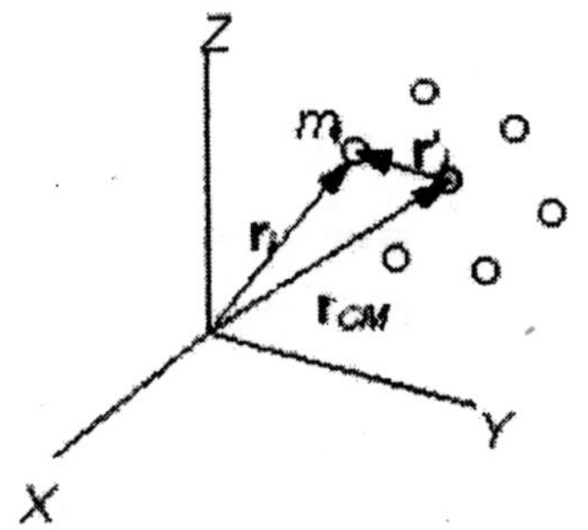

Figure 3

$$\mathbf{r}_i = \mathbf{r}_{CM} + \mathbf{r}'_i$$

$$\mathbf{q} = \sum_i m_i \mathbf{r}_i = \sum_i m_i (\mathbf{r}_{CM} + \mathbf{r}'_i)$$

$$= \sum_i m_i \mathbf{r}_{CM} + \sum_i m_i \mathbf{r}'_i$$

$$= \left(\sum_i m_i \right) \mathbf{r}_{CM} + \sum_i m_i \mathbf{r}'_i \quad [5]$$

The second term of [5] is the total 1st mass moment of the system with respect to its CM. From [3] and [5]:

$$\sum_i m_i \mathbf{r}'_i = 0 \quad [6]$$

In other words, the sum of the 1st mass moments of the particles with respect to their CM always becomes zero.

In Figure 1, the velocity of particle *i* can be expressed as

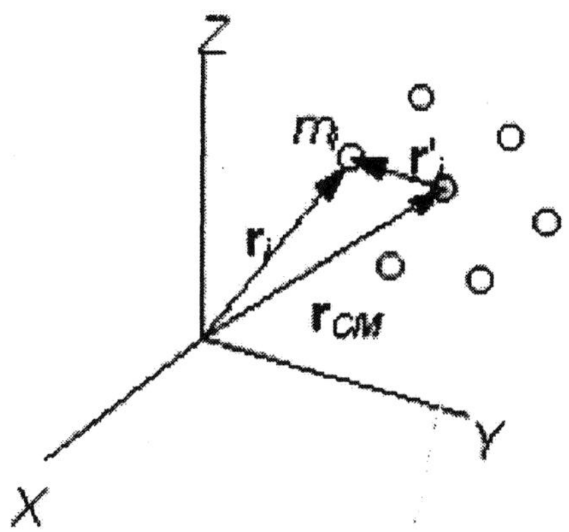

Figure 1

$$\mathbf{v}_i = \frac{d\mathbf{r}_i}{dt} = \frac{d}{dt}(\mathbf{r}_{CM} + \mathbf{r}'_i)$$
$$= \mathbf{v}_{CM} + \mathbf{v}'_i \qquad [1]$$

Using [3] of Linear Kinetics-Particle, one can express the momentum of the system as

$$\mathbf{p} = \sum_i \mathbf{p}_i = \sum_i m_i \mathbf{v}_i = \sum_i m_i (\mathbf{v}_{CM} + \mathbf{v}'_i)$$
$$= \sum_i m_i \mathbf{v}_{CM} + \sum_i m_i \mathbf{v}'_i$$
$$= \left(\sum_i m_i\right) \cdot \mathbf{v}_{CM} + \sum_i m_i \mathbf{v}'_i$$
$$= m_{total} \cdot \mathbf{v}_{CM} \qquad [2]$$

since, from [6] of Center of Mass-System of Particles,

$$\sum_i m_i \mathbf{v}'_i = \sum_i \left(m_i \frac{d\mathbf{r}'_i}{dt} \right)$$
$$= \frac{d}{dt}\left(\sum_i m_i \mathbf{r}'_i \right)$$
$$= 0 \qquad [3]$$

As shown in [2], the momentum of a system of particles is simply equal to that of its CM.

Rigid Body Dynamics

For analytical convenience, human body segments are considered as rigid bodies. A rigid body is similar to a system of particles in the sense that it is composed of particles.

Therefore most of the equations for a system of particles are usable in the dynamics of a rigid body. The main difference is of course that the rigid body is **rigid**. There is no migration of mass within a rigid body. As a result, the relative positions among the particles composing a rigid body do not change. This will further simplify the equations obtained from a system of particles.

The main strategy in analyzing the motion of a rigid body is to split the motion into the linear motion of the CM and the angular motion of the body about its CM. This is because all particles composing the body show the same relative angular motion about the CM.

In other words, one can describe the motion of the rigid body as a whole rather than those of the particles individually. The physical characteristics of a rigid body can be described by its inertial properties: mass and moment of inertia. For this reason, a major portion of discussion will be dedicated to the inertial properties of the rigid body: moment of inertia & inertia tensor.

The pages included in this section are:

- Moment of Inertia
- Calculation of the MOI
- Inertia Tensor
- Principal Axes
- Transformation of the Inertia Tensor
- Angular Momentum
- Kinetic Energy

The rigid body dynamics will serve as the building blocks for a more complex type of motion later: motion of a system of rigid bodies.

Moment of Inertia of Systems of Particles

Newton's first law of motion says "A body maintains the current state of motion unless acted upon by an external force." The measure of the inertia in the linear motion is the **mass** of the system and its angular counterpart is the so-called **moment of inertia**.

The moment of inertia of a body is not only related to its mass but also the distribution of the mass throughout the body. So two bodies of the same mass may possess different moments of inertia.

A rigid body can be considered as a system of particles in which the relative positions of the particles do not change. The moment of inertia of a single particle (*I*) can be expressed as

$$I = mr^2 \quad [1]$$

where *m* = the mass of the particle, and *r* = the shortest distance from the axis of rotation to the particle (Figure 1).

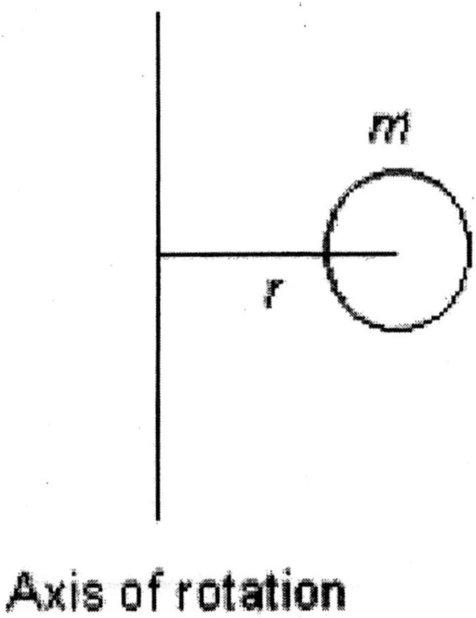

Figure 1

As shown in [1], moment of inertia is equal to mass times square of the distance and it is also referred to as **the second mass moment**.

Mass times distance, *m***r**, is called as **the first mass moment**. This concept of first mass moment is normally used in deriving the center of mass of a system of particles or a rigid body. See Center of Mass-System of Particles for the details.

Expanding [1] for a system of particles:

$$I = \sum_i m_i r_i^2 \quad [2]$$

Moment of Inertia of a Rigid Body

Based on [2], one can obtain the moment of inertia of a rigid by shown in Figure 2:

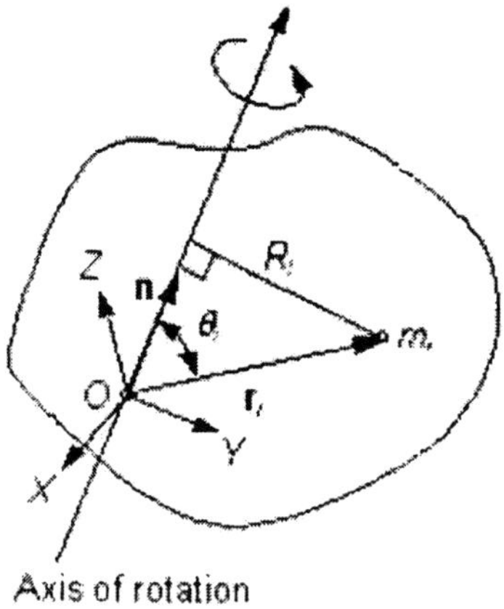

Figure 2

$$
\begin{aligned}
I &= \sum_i m_i R_i^2 \\
&= \sum_i m_i \left(|\mathbf{r}_i| \sin\theta_i \right)^2 \\
&= \sum_i m_i |\mathbf{r}_i \times \mathbf{n}|^2 \\
&= \sum_i m_i (\mathbf{r}_i \times \mathbf{n}) \cdot (\mathbf{r}_i \times \mathbf{n})
\end{aligned} \qquad [3]
$$

where $\mathbf{r}_i$ = the position of particle i, and $\mathbf{n}$ = the unit vector of the axis of rotation. Note here that the axis of rotation passes through the local reference frame, the *OXYZ* system. Let

$$\mathbf{r}_i = x_i\mathbf{i} + y_i\mathbf{j} + z_i\mathbf{k} = \begin{bmatrix} x_i \\ y_i \\ z_i \end{bmatrix} \qquad [4]$$

and

$$\mathbf{n} = \cos\alpha\mathbf{i} + \cos\beta\mathbf{j} + \cos\gamma\mathbf{k} = \begin{bmatrix} \cos\alpha \\ \cos\beta \\ \cos\gamma \end{bmatrix} \qquad [5]$$

where $\cos\alpha$, $\cos\beta$ & $\cos\gamma$ = the three direction cosines of vector **n** to the *XYZ* system. Substituting [4] & [5] into [3] leads to

$$I = \sum_i m_i(\mathbf{r}_i \times \mathbf{n})\cdot(\mathbf{r}_i \times \mathbf{n})$$

$$= \sum_i m_i \left[\begin{bmatrix} 0 & -z_i & y_i \\ z_i & 0 & -x_i \\ -y_i & x_i & 0 \end{bmatrix}\begin{bmatrix}\cos\alpha \\ \cos\beta \\ \cos\gamma\end{bmatrix}\right]^t \left[\begin{bmatrix} 0 & -z_i & y_i \\ z_i & 0 & -x_i \\ -y_i & x_i & 0 \end{bmatrix}\begin{bmatrix}\cos\alpha \\ \cos\beta \\ \cos\gamma\end{bmatrix}\right]$$

$$= \sum_i m_i \begin{bmatrix} y_i\cos\gamma - z_i\cos\beta \\ z_i\cos\alpha - x_i\cos\gamma \\ x_i\cos\beta - y_i\cos\alpha \end{bmatrix}^t \begin{bmatrix} y_i\cos\gamma - z_i\cos\beta \\ z_i\cos\alpha - x_i\cos\gamma \\ x_i\cos\beta - y_i\cos\alpha \end{bmatrix}$$

$$= \sum_i m_i\left[(y_i\cos\gamma - z_i\cos\beta)^2 + (z_i\cos\alpha - x_i\cos\gamma)^2 + (x_i\cos\beta - y_i\cos\alpha)^2\right]$$

$$= I_{xx}\cos^2\alpha + I_{yy}\cos^2\beta + I_{zz}\cos^2\gamma + 2I_{xy}\cos\alpha\cos\beta + 2I_{yz}\cos\beta\cos\gamma + 2I_{zx}\cos\gamma\cos\alpha$$

[6]

where

$$I_{xx} \equiv \sum_i m_i(y_i^2 + z_i^2) \quad I_{yy} \equiv \sum_i m_i(z_i^2 + x_i^2) \quad I_{zz} \equiv \sum_i m_i(x_i^2 + y_i^2)$$

$$I_{xy} = I_{yx} \equiv -\sum_i m_i x_i y_i$$

$$I_{xz} = I_{zx} \equiv -\sum_i m_i x_i z_i$$

$$I_{yz} = I_{zy} \equiv -\sum_i m_i y_i z_i$$

[7]

I_{xx}, I_{yy} & I_{zz} are called the **moments of inertia** while I_{xy}, I_{yx}, I_{yz}, I_{zy}, I_{zx}, & I_{xz} are the **products of inertia**. For a rigid body, the relative position of the particles do not change and one can write [7] as:

$$I_{xx} = \int (y^2 + z^2) \cdot dm \quad I_{yy} = \int (z^2 + x^2) \cdot dm \quad I_{zz} = \int (x^2 + y^2) \cdot dm$$

$$I_{xy} = I_{yx} = -\int xy \cdot dm$$

$$I_{xz} = I_{zx} = -\int xz \cdot dm$$

$$I_{yz} = I_{zy} = -\int yz \cdot dm$$

[8]

When the shape and the density distribution of the rigid body is precisely known, one can use [8] to compute the moments and products of inertia. (See BSP Equations for the MOI equations of the typical geometric shapes commonly used in human body modeling.)

Otherwise, it is difficult to compute them through integration. Rather, the moment of inertia must be measured directly from the object. See Measuring MOI for the details.

Ellipsoid of Inertia

The moments and products of inertia shown in [7] and [8] are basically specific to the local reference frame defined and reflect the mass distribution within the body in relation to the local reference frame.

As shown in [6], the actual moment of inertia of a rigid body about an axis of rotation is a function of not only the moments and products of inertia for a given reference frame but also the orientation of the axis of rotation, α, β & γ.

Thus, it would be more accurate to say that the moment of inertia of a rigid body reflects the mass distribution within the body with respect to the axis of rotation.

As the axis of rotation changes, so does the moment of inertia. To show this point clearly, let

$$u \equiv \frac{1}{\sqrt{I}} \cos\alpha \quad v \equiv \frac{1}{\sqrt{I}} \cos\beta \quad w \equiv \frac{1}{\sqrt{I}} \cos\gamma \qquad [9]$$

Substituting [9] into [6] yields

$$I_{xx}u^2 + I_{yy}v^2 + I_{zz}w^2 + 2I_{xy}uv + 2I_{yz}vw + 2I_{zx}wx = 1 \qquad [10]$$

Interestingly, [10] suffices the general form of the **ellipsoid** with its center at the origin of the reference frame. When $I_{xy} = I_{yz} = I_{zx} = 0$, the ellipsoid defined by [10] definitely becomes symmetric about the three axes.

Since

$$u^2 + v^2 + w^2 = \frac{1}{I} \qquad [11]$$

the distance from the center of the ellipsoid to the surface is 1 divided by the square root of the moment of inertia of the rigid body for a given orientation, α, β & γ. The ellipsoid defined by [10] is called **the ellipsoid of inertia** since it describes the moment of inertia of an object as a function of the orientation of the axis of rotation.

Calculation of the MOI

In computation of the moment of inertia, one can replace the summation shown in [2] of Inertia Tensor by an integration over the body:

$$I = \int r^2 \cdot dm \qquad [1]$$

where r = the perpendicular distance from the particle to the axis of rotation, and dm = the mass of the particle which is a function of the density.

Thin Rod

Let's now apply [1] to a thin uniform rod shown in Figure 1. The MOI of the rod about the Y axis is

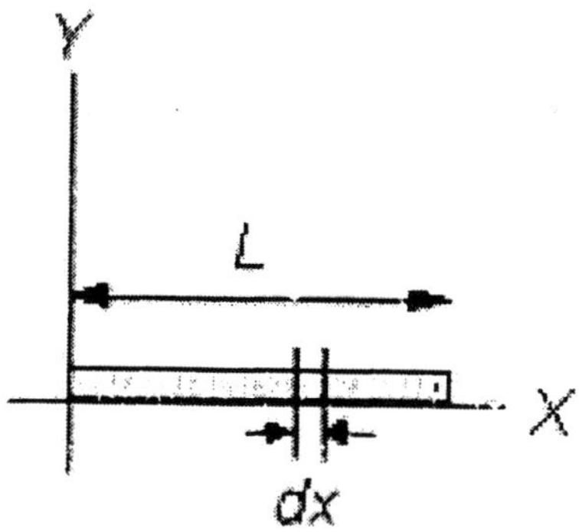

Figure 1

$$I_y = \int_0^L r^2 \cdot dm = \int_0^L x^2 (\rho \cdot dx)$$

$$= \rho \int_0^L x^2 \quad [illegible] \quad \lfloor_0 \quad [illegible] \quad \frac{1}{3} mL^2$$

[2]

since

$$dm = \rho \cdot dx$$

$$m = \rho L$$

[3]

where ρ = the density of the rod, m = the mass of the rod, and L = the length of the rod.

Circular Ring

The moment of inertia of the uniform circular ring shown in Figure 2 about the *Z* axis (the symmetry axis) is

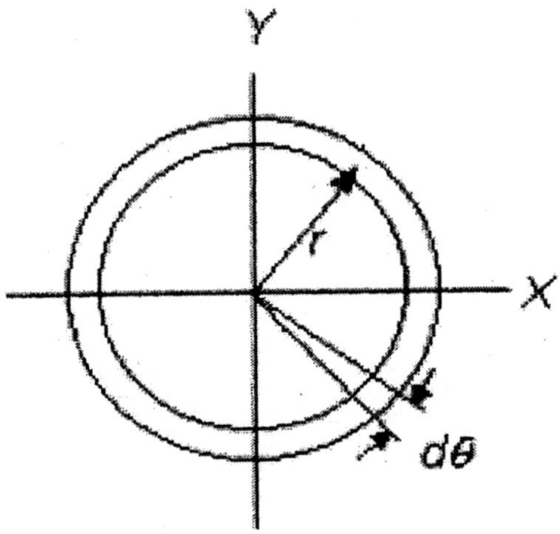

Figure 2

$$I_{zz} = \int_0^{2\pi} r^2 \cdot dm = \int_0^{2\pi} r^2(\rho \cdot dl)$$

$$= \int_0^{2\pi} r^2(\rho r \cdot d\theta) = \rho r^3 \int_0^{2\pi} d\theta = 2\pi\rho r^3 = mr^2 \quad [4]$$

since

$$dm = \rho \cdot dl$$
$$dl = r \cdot d\theta$$
$$m = 2\pi\rho r \quad [5]$$

where dl = the length of the arc formed by $d\theta$. [5] is also applicable to a circular cylinder.

Circular Disc

A uniform circular disc of radius R can be considered as a cascade of uniform circular rings as shown in Figure 3. Thus, from [5], the moment of inertia about the Z axis (the symmetry axis) becomes

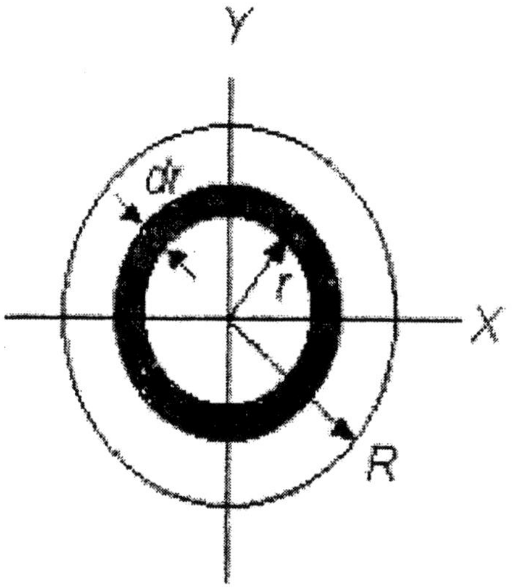

Figure 3

$$I_{zz} = \int_0^R 2\pi\rho r^3 \cdot dr$$

$$= 2\pi\rho\left[\frac{r^4}{4}\right]_0^R = \frac{1}{2}\pi\rho R^4 = \frac{1}{2}mR^2 \quad [6]$$

since

$$m = \pi R^2 \quad [7]$$

[6] can be used in computing the MOI of a circular bar about its longitudinal axis as well.

Sphere

A uniform sphere can be considered as a cascade of uniform circular discs as shown in Figure 4. From [6], the moment of inertia about the vertical axis (*Z* axis) is

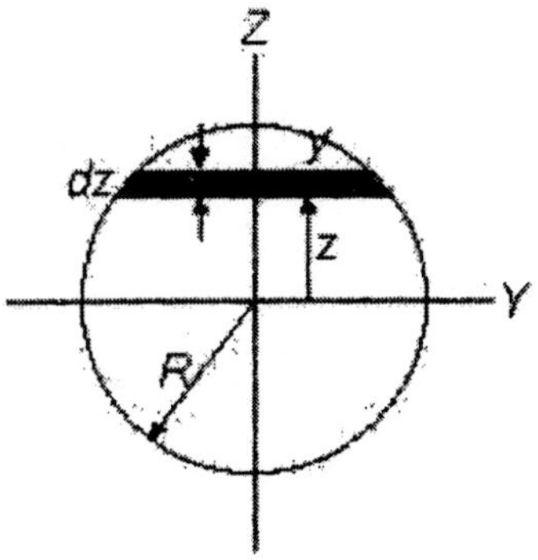

Figure 4

$$I_{zz} = \int_{-R}^{R}\left[\frac{1}{2}\pi\rho y^4\right]\cdot dz$$

$$= \int_{-R}^{R}\left[\frac{1}{2}\pi\rho\left(R^2 - z^2\right)^2\right]\cdot dz = \frac{1}{2}\pi\rho\int_{-R}^{R}\left[R^4 - 2R^2z^2 + z^4\right]\cdot dz$$

$$= \frac{1}{2}\pi\rho\left[R^4z - \frac{2}{3}R^2z^3 + \frac{1}{5}z^5\right]_{-R}^{R} = \frac{8}{15}\pi\rho R^5 = \frac{2}{5}mR^2 \quad [8]$$

since

$$m = \frac{4}{3}\pi\rho R^3 \quad [9]$$

See BSP Equations for the moment-of-inertia equations for the geometric shapes commonly used in the human body modeling.

Perpendicular-Axis Theorem

Now, let's go back to the uniform circular disc (Figure 3). The moment of inertia of a uniform circular disc about its perpendicular axis (Z axis) can be expressed as

$$\begin{aligned} I_{zz} &= \sum_i m_i r_i^2 = \sum_i m_i\left(x_i^2 + y_i^2\right) \\ &= \sum_i m_i x_i^2 + \sum_i m_i y_i^2 \\ &= I_{yy} + I_{xx} = I_{xx} + I_{yy} \end{aligned} \qquad [10]$$

since

$$\begin{aligned} I_{xx} &= \sum_i m_i y_i^2 \\ I_{yy} &= \sum_i m_i x_i^2 \end{aligned} \qquad [11]$$

In other words, the MOI about the Z axis is equal to sum of those about the X and Y axes. [10] is true for any rigid lamina: the MOI of any rigid lamina about an axis normal to the lamina plane is equal to the sum of the MOIs about any two perpendicular axes lying on the plane and passing through the normal axis. This is the so-called **perpendicular-axis theorem**.

Since the circular disc has symmetric shape,

$$I_{xx} = I_{yy} \qquad [12]$$

and, from [6]:

$$\begin{aligned} I_{xx} &= I_{yy} = \frac{I_{zz}}{2} \\ &= \frac{1}{4}\pi\rho R^4 = \frac{1}{4} m R^2 \end{aligned} \qquad [13]$$

One can directly obtain [13] from [11] or

$$I_{xx} = \int y_i^2 \cdot dm$$
$$I_{yy} = \int x_i^2 \cdot dm \quad [14]$$

[2] can be used in further developing [14] to obtain [13]. See BSP Equations for this approach.

Parallel-Axis Theorem

Now, let's compute the MOI of a uniform circular column. Circular bar can be regarded as a cascade of circular discs as shown in Figure 5. From [13]:

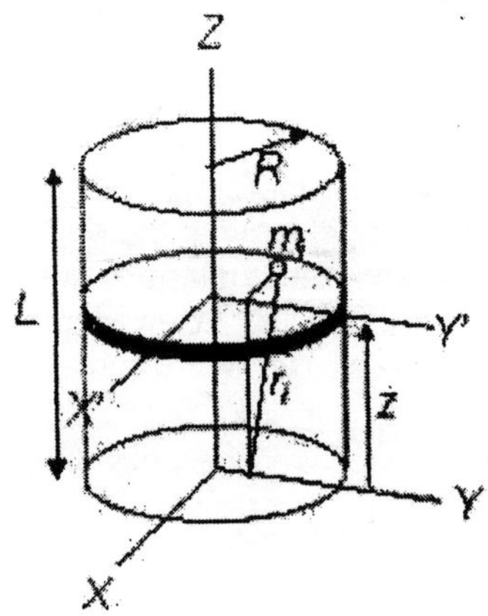

Figure 5

$$I_{yy}(disc) = \sum_i m_i \cdot r_i^2 = \sum_i m_i \cdot (x_i^2 + z^2) = \sum_i m_i \cdot x_i^2 + \left[\sum_i m_i\right] \cdot z^2$$
$$= \sum_i m_i \cdot x_i^2 + m_{disc} \cdot z^2 = I_{y'y'}(disc) + m_{disc} \cdot z^2$$
$$= \frac{1}{4}\pi\rho R^4 + \pi\rho R^2 z^2$$

[15]

since

$$m_{disc} = \pi\rho R^2$$
$$I_{y'y'}(disc) = \frac{1}{4}\pi\rho R^4 \quad [16]$$

where m_{disc} = mass of the circular disc, and $I_{y'y'}$(disc) = the MOI of the disc about the *Y'* axis. [16] basically says that the MOI of a circular plate about the *Y* axis is equal to the sum of the MOI about the parallel axis on the disc (*Y'*) and the mass of the disc times square of the distance between the two axes. This is the so-called **parallel-axis theorem**.

The MOI of the circular column is therefore

$$I_{yy} = \int_0^L I_{yy}(disc)\cdot dz = \int_0^L\left[\frac{1}{4}\pi\rho R^4 + \pi\rho R^2 z^2\right]\cdot dz = \int_0^L\left[\frac{1}{4}\pi\rho R^4\right]\cdot dz + \int_0^L\left[\pi\rho R^2 z^2\right]\cdot dz$$
$$= \frac{1}{4}\pi\rho R^4\left[z\right]_0^L + \pi\rho R^2\left[\frac{z^3}{3}\right]_0^L = \frac{1}{4}\pi\rho R^4 L + \frac{1}{3}\pi\rho R^2 L^3$$
$$= \pi\rho R^2 L\left[\frac{1}{4}R^2 + \frac{1}{3}L^2\right] = m\left[\frac{1}{4}R^2 + \frac{1}{3}L^2\right]$$

[17]

since

$$m = \pi\rho R^2 L \quad [18]$$

Comparing [18] with [2], one can clearly see the difference in the MOI between a thin rod and a thick rod (circular column). Similarly, [13] and [17] shows the difference in the MOI between a circular disc and a thick circular plate (circular column).

Physical Pendulum & Direct Measurement

Unfortunately, the integration approach is possible only when the body has a known geometric shape. In the mathematical human body models such as *Hanavan (1964)* and *Yeadon (1990)*, it is assumed that the body segments show a group of geometric shapes such as ellipsoid of revolution, elliptical solids, and stadium solids. See BSP Equations for the details.

If the body has a irregular shape, the integration approach has not much use and a direct measurement must be attempted. Figure 6 shows a body with irregular shape which is rotating freely about an axis passing through its one end. The *X* axis is the axis of rotation, thus, the center of mass (CM) of the body moves within the *YZ* plane.

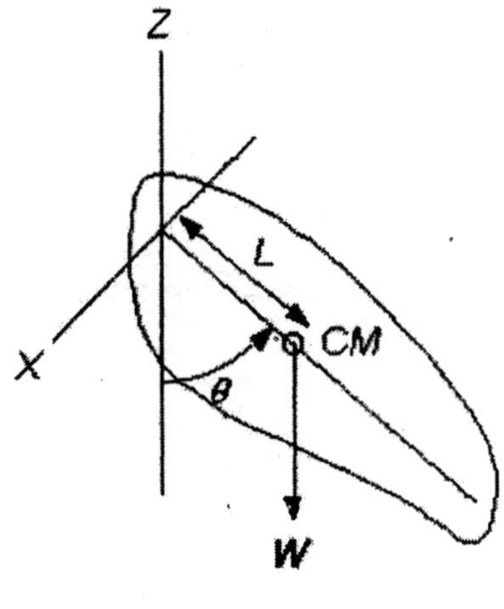

Figure 6

The torque produced by the weight of the body about the *X* axis is then

$$T_x = I_{xx}\alpha = mgL \cdot \sin\theta \quad [19]$$

where T_x = the torque about the *X* axis, I_{xx} = MOI of the body about the *X* axis, α = angular acceleration, m = the mass of the body, g = the gravitational acceleration (9.81 m/s^2), and L = the distance between the axis of rotation to the body's CM. For a small θ,

$\sin\theta \approx \theta$ **[20]**

and, from [19],

$I_{xx}\ddot{\theta} + mgL\theta = 0$ **[21]**

Solving [21] for θ, one obtains

$$\theta = \theta_0 \cdot \cos(2\pi ft - \varepsilon)$$

$$f = \frac{1}{2\pi}\sqrt{\frac{mgL}{I_{xx}}}$$

$$T = \frac{1}{f} = 2\pi\sqrt{\frac{I_{xx}}{mgL}}$$

$$T^2 = 4\pi^2 \frac{I_{xx}}{mgL}$$

$$I_{xx} = \frac{T^2}{4\pi^2} mgL$$

[22]

where θ_o = the amplitude, f = the frequency of the pendulum, ε = the phase angle, T = the period of the pendulum. As shown in [22], the MOI of the body about the X axis, after all, can be computed from the period of a small pendulum motion of the body. The MOI about the parallel axis, which passes through the CM of the body, can be also computed based on the parallel-axis theorem:

$I_{CMxx} = I_{xx} - mL^2$ **[23]**

Principal Moments of inertia

As shown in [6] in Inertia Tensor, the angular momentum of a rigid body with respect to the origin of the local reference frame is expressed as

$$\mathbf{H}=\begin{bmatrix} I_{xx} & I_{xy} & I_{xz} \\ I_{yx} & I_{yy} & I_{yz} \\ I_{zx} & I_{zy} & I_{zz} \end{bmatrix}\begin{bmatrix} \omega_x \\ \omega_y \\ \omega_z \end{bmatrix}=\begin{bmatrix} I_{xx}\omega_x+I_{xy}\omega_y+I_{xz}\omega_z \\ I_{yx}\omega_x+I_{yy}\omega_y+I_{yz}\omega_z \\ I_{zx}\omega_x+I_{zy}\omega_y+I_{zz}\omega_z \end{bmatrix} \quad [1]$$

If, by chance, all the off-diagonal terms of the inertia tensor shown in [1] become zero, [1] can be further simplified to

$$\mathbf{H}=\begin{bmatrix} I_{xx} & 0 & 0 \\ 0 & I_{yy} & 0 \\ 0 & 0 & I_{zz} \end{bmatrix}\begin{bmatrix} \omega_x \\ \omega_y \\ \omega_z \end{bmatrix}=\begin{bmatrix} I_{xx}\omega_x \\ I_{yy}\omega_y \\ I_{zz}\omega_z \end{bmatrix} \quad [2]$$

This can happen when one aligns the axes of the local reference frame in such a way that the mass of the body evenly distribute around the axes, thus, the product-of-inertia terms all vanish. The non-zero diagonal terms of the inertia tensor shown in [2] are called **the principal moments of inertia** of the object.

Principal Axes

As shown in [1], there is no guarantee that the angular momentum vector has the same direction to that of the angular velocity vector. This causes a problem: if the direction of the angular momentum keeps changing, it develops a torque which eventually forces the axis of rotation to move. This is the main reason that causes wearing and vibration in machinery with rotating parts.

But in some special cases, the following condition may hold so that the angular momentum and velocity vectors show the same direction:

$$\mathbf{H}=\begin{bmatrix} I_{xx} & I_{xy} & I_{xz} \\ I_{yx} & I_{yy} & I_{yz} \\ I_{zx} & I_{zy} & I_{zz} \end{bmatrix}\boldsymbol{\omega}=I\boldsymbol{\omega} \quad [3]$$

where I = the equivalent scalar moment of inertia of the body about the axis of rotation. Any axis of rotation of the body which suffices [3] is called a **principal axis**. There are a group of principal axes (theoretically 3) in a three-dimensional body. For example, there are three perpendicular principal axes for the system shown in Figure 1.

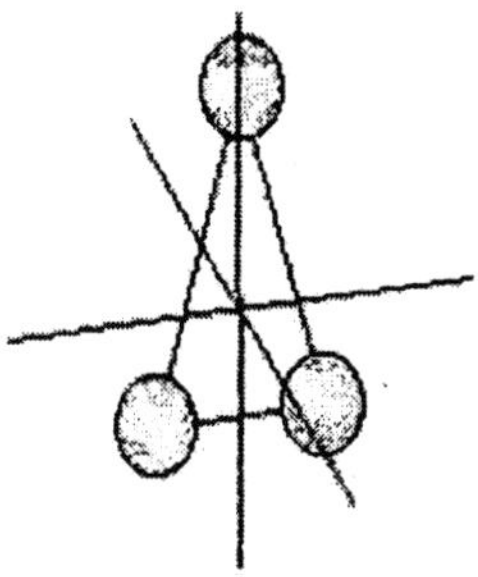

Figure 1

[3] basically says that the inertia tensor can be replaced with a single scalar moment of inertia when the axis of rotation is a principal axis.

Diagonalization of the Inertia Tensor

From [3]:

$$\begin{bmatrix} I_{xx} & I_{xy} & I_{xz} \\ I_{yx} & I_{yy} & I_{yz} \\ I_{zx} & I_{zy} & I_{zz} \end{bmatrix} \boldsymbol{\omega} = I\boldsymbol{\omega}$$

$$\begin{bmatrix} I_{xx} & I_{xy} & I_{xz} \\ I_{yx} & I_{yy} & I_{yz} \\ I_{zx} & I_{zy} & I_{zz} \end{bmatrix} \boldsymbol{\omega} - I\boldsymbol{\omega} = \begin{bmatrix} I_{xx} & I_{xy} & I_{xz} \\ I_{yx} & I_{yy} & I_{yz} \\ I_{zx} & I_{zy} & I_{zz} \end{bmatrix} \boldsymbol{\omega} - I\begin{bmatrix} 1 & 0 & 0 \\ 0 & 1 & 0 \\ 0 & 0 & 1 \end{bmatrix} \boldsymbol{\omega}$$

$$= \begin{bmatrix} I_{xx} - I & I_{xy} & I_{xz} \\ I_{yx} & I_{yy} - I & I_{yz} \\ I_{zx} & I_{zy} & I_{zz} - I \end{bmatrix} \boldsymbol{\omega} = 0 \qquad [4]$$

Or [4] can be simplified to

$$[\mathbf{I} - I\mathbf{1}]\boldsymbol{\omega} = 0 \qquad [5]$$

where **1** = the identity matrix. *I* shown in [5] is called an eigenvalue while ω is the eigenvector. [5] is the eigenvalue equation.

In order for [5] to have a nontrivial solution the determinant of the coefficients should vanish:

$$\begin{vmatrix} I_{xx} - I & I_{xy} & I_{xz} \\ I_{yx} & I_{yy} - I & I_{yz} \\ I_{zx} & I_{zy} & I_{zz} - I \end{vmatrix} = 0 \qquad [6]$$

[6] leads to the **secular equation** which is basically cubic, thus provides three roots (eigenvalues): I_1, I_2 & I_3. Each root corresponds to a moment of inertia about a principal axis. In fact the three roots are the principal moments of inertia of the rigid body introduced in [2]:

$$\mathbf{I} = \begin{bmatrix} I_1 & 0 & 0 \\ 0 & I_2 & 0 \\ 0 & 0 & I_3 \end{bmatrix} \qquad [7]$$

Once the eigenvalues are known, the principal axes can be computed. Let

$$\mathbf{n} \equiv \begin{bmatrix} n_x \\ n_y \\ n_z \end{bmatrix} \qquad [8]$$

where **n** = the unit vector of the principal axis, thus,

$$n_x^2 + n_y^2 + n_z^2 = 1 \qquad [9]$$

From [4] & [8]:

$$\begin{bmatrix} I_{xx}-I & I_{xy} & I_{xz} \\ I_{yx} & I_{yy}-I & I_{yz} \\ I_{zx} & I_{zy} & I_{zz}-I \end{bmatrix} \begin{bmatrix} n_x \\ n_y \\ n_z \end{bmatrix} = 0$$

$$(I_{xx}-I)n_x + I_{xy}n_y + I_{xz}n_z = 0$$
$$I_{yx}n_x + (I_{yy}-I)n_y + I_{yz}n_z = 0$$
$$I_{zx}n_x + I_{zy}n_y + (I_{zz}-I)n_z = 0 \quad [10]$$

For each eigenvalue, one can compute the corresponding n_x, n_y & n_z from [9] & [10]. One must pay attention to the direction of the eigenvector in this process.

In motion analysis, the principal moments of inertia can be obtained from the inertial properties of the body segments. I_1, I_2 & I_3 of each segment are generally known. The data are available in the form of the radius-of-gyration ratios (ratio of the radius of gyration to the segment length), regression equations, and scaling coefficients. One can also compute the principal moments of inertia of the body segments through modeling using some geometric shapes.

Projectile Motion

In many sport activities the performer moves freely through the air. Diving, gymnastics, high jumping, long jumping and figure skating are a few examples where such motion occurs. In addition, sports implements are projected in events like the shot-put, discus, baseball and soccer. In both situations, the motion is that of a "projectile" and is controlled by well understood physical laws.

Once the projectile (either performer or projected object) is in the air, only two external forces act upon it. The first is the force of gravity acting vertically and the second is due to air drag effects acting in a direction primarily opposite to the direction of motion. The latter force is an important factor in such sports as ski-jumping and skydiving because the velocity is quite high and the flight time is quite long. It is also of special significance in the javelin and discus events because of the aerodynamic characteristics of the implements involved. However, in many activities involving projectile motion air resistance plays an insignificant role. Because of this and in order to simplify the following calculations, we will neglect the air resistance forces that are involved. We will assume such forces to be zero.

Force Measurement

- In this lab the focus of study is vertical ground reaction force (GRF) and subsequent vertical motion of the body. Reaction Forces are equal and opposite to the forces applied by the body to the ground (Newton's 3rd law). In addition, Newton's 2nd law (F = m a) governs the resulting motion.

  A force platform is a device which measures ground reaction force. It is a three dimensional measuring device, however we will deal only with the vertical component of the ground reaction force. A free body diagram of the plate and a subject is illustrated below:

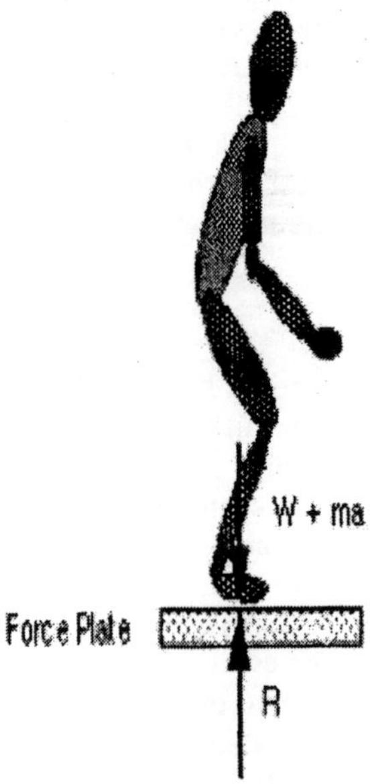

$$F = ma$$
$$F = R - W$$
$$ma = R - W$$
$$R = W + ma$$

where W is weight of subject, R is reaction force, m is mass of subject and a is acceleration of subject.

For the case in which a person is stationary on the plate, the two forces (W and R) must be equal in magnitude and opposite in direction. If the person starts to move upward (acceleration of CM is positive), then ma is positive and the ground reaction force will increase in magnitude. With initiation of a downwards movement (negative acceleration of the CM), ma is negative and the ground reaction force will decrease below body weight.

In summary:

- **if acceleration is less than 0 then R is less than W**
- **if acceleration = 0 then R = W**
- **if acceleration is greater than 0 then R is greater than W**

- **Procedures**

Each student will perform the following jumps on the force platform while it monitors the vertical ground reaction force:

1. With hands on hips from a squat position, perform a maximal vertical jump **without counter movement.**
2. With hands on hips from an upright position, perform a maximal vertical jump **with counter movement.**

During each jump, ***keep your hands on your hips throughout the jump****. When you land, stand up but do not step off the force plate until directed to do so. You will receive a force-time file on disk for each jump. Do* ***not*** *attach the force-time data sheet to your lab after graphing the data.*

- **Results**

Each member of the group should perform a "zero" correction to their data so that the GRF when airborne is zero. Then use the graphing capabilities of the spreadsheet to graph force versus time for each jump for ONE member of your lab group.

Manually label the graphs with the following:

0. Body Weight line
1. Takeoff (TO)
2. Landing (L)
3. Flight Time (FT)

Impulse and Ground Reaction Force

- In last week's lab, you measured the vertical ground reaction force during vertical jumps. The force-time curves which resulted were assessed qualitatively without detailing the relationships of force to resulting movement. This week's lab will continue with analysis of ground reaction forces (GRF) and the relationship of force, time, impulse and velocity.

Newton's second law (F = ma) can be written in a form which includes the definition of acceleration:

$$F = m\frac{\Delta V}{\Delta t}$$

With simple algebraic rearrangement, this can be written as:

$$F\ \Delta t = m\Delta V$$

or

Impulse = Change of Momentum

The "Impulse" part of this expression is a new quantity in our study of mechanics. It depends on both force and the time over which the force was applied. Units of impulse involve force and time: N*s.

This impulse-momentum relationship is an important means of determining what motion results from an applied force. In the case of constant force application, impulse is particularly easy to calculate. However, if force is not constant (which is typical of most real situations) a slightly different understanding must be used. Consider the force-time graphs shown in figure.

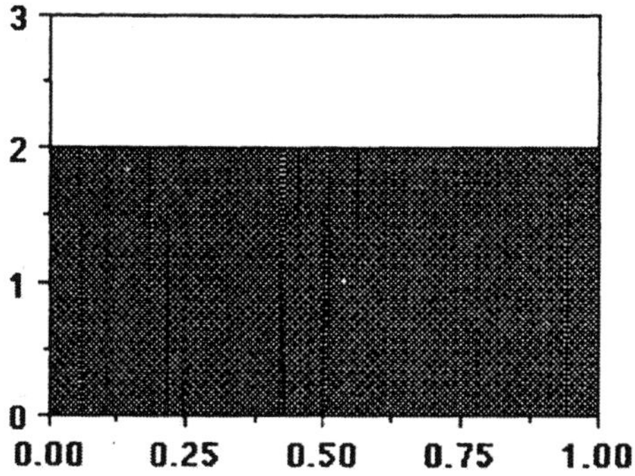

Time in seconds

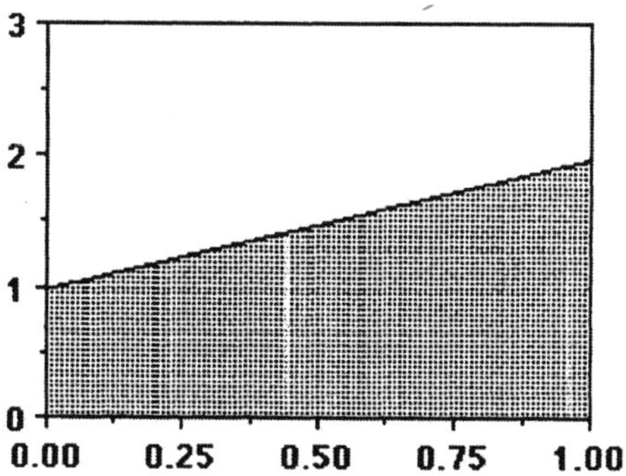

Time in seconds

In the first graph, force is constant. The impulse of the force is just the value of the force times the time of application. On the graph, this corresponds to the shaded rectangular area below the force line (2 Ns).

On the second graph, force is not constant. The impulse cannot be calculated based on a constant force times its period of application as was done in the first case. However, the idea of area under the force graph is still appropriate. If we could determine that area we would know the impulse (and consequently the change of momentum).

So, how to determine the area under the force-time graph? Several ways of estimating the area under a graph are often used:

1. Plot the graph on a grid and count the number of squares under the curve.
2. Approximate the force-time curve using straight line segments. Then use formulas for the area of triangles and rectangles.
3. Approximate the area as a set of vertical bars where the height of each bar is the average values of the data points at sides of the bar. The area of each bar (a rectangle) is then the product of its height and its width (time between measurements). The impulse is the sum of the areas of the bars.

This is illustrated below for forces of 1, 1.2, 1.5, 1.9, 2.4 and 3.0 N at the times **shown on the graph.** The impulse of the first shaded bar can be found by first getting the average force of the two samples determining its height (1.2 and 1.5 N). The average force is 1.35 N over the interval of 0.2 seconds (0.2 to 0.4). Hence the impulse (shaded area) is 1.35 N times 0.2 seconds which is 0.27 Ns.

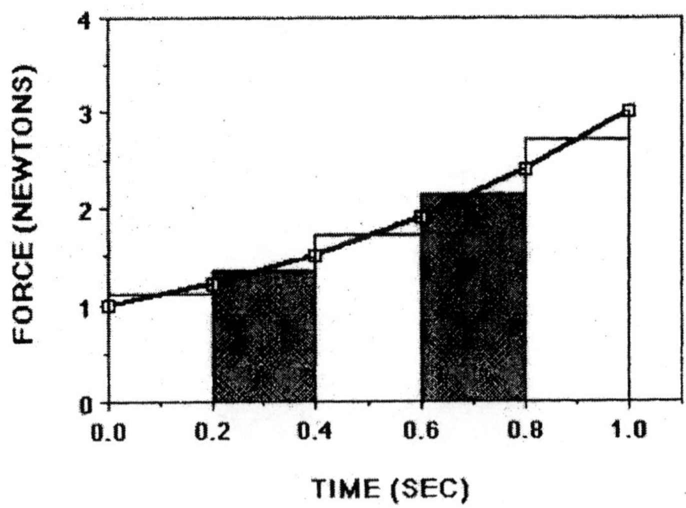

For the second shaded bar the average force is 2.15 N and the impulse would be 0.43 Ns of impulse. If you follow this procedure for the whole area under these six data points, the impulse is 1.8 Ns.

In general, this third method is most commonly used in determining the impulse of biomechanical forces.

- **Part 1 Methods**

A **vertical jump force-time curve** has been included for illustration. A body weight (BW) line has been added to the graph. The total force acting on the jumper is the ground reaction force minus gravitational force (BW). Thus to calculate the impulse, one must first subtract off body weight. In effect, this is as if the zero point for the force axis was shifted upward. The shaded regions of the graph sum to produce the impulse before takeoff and the impulse after landing. The regions below the BW line are "negative areas."

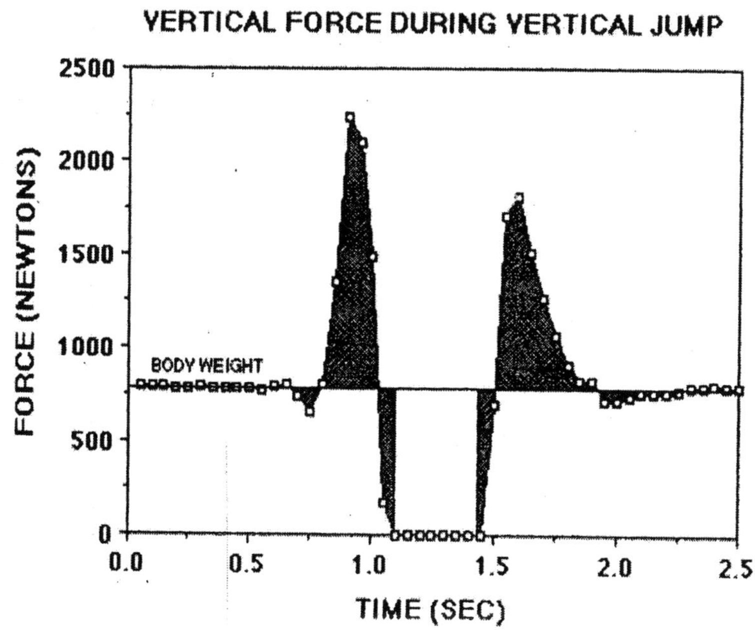

In equation form this can be written out as follows:

First, let Fi be the force at some instant in time. The total force acting on the person at that instant will be Fi - Body Weight (BW). The impulse of the force for samples Fi and Fi+1 would be:

$$\text{Impulse} = \frac{(F_i - BW) + (F_{i+1} - BW)}{2} * (\text{Time Interval between samples})$$

Note that this is the area or Impulse under just one strip or one interval from i to i+1. The Total Impulse would involve summing each of these strips up to the time of takeoff.

To determine body weight (BW), take an average force from the first several (20-30) frames of "zero corrected" data. This average is the Body Weight (don't worry that it doesn't match your body weight precisely).

Using force-time data from last week's lab, determine the vertical impulse up to the point of takeoff for both of your jumps (Squat & Countermovement). Then determine the impulse from the landing point in time to the end of the data collection. Use a spreadsheet to calculate the total impulse. Set up the spreadsheet as follows:

Time (seconds)	**GRF (N)**	**GRF - BW (N)**	**Average Force (N)**	**Area of strip (N*s)**
0.00				
0.01				
0.02				
0.03				
0.04				
etc.				

In your spreadsheet, write a formula to determine the impulse up to takeoff and the impulse from the landing point. Make note of the flight time of the jump.

- **Part 2 Methods**

On an attached page, Force-Time data are tabulated along with a graph to illustrate the characteristics of a **standing long jump**. Determine the **vertical and horizontal impulse** for the jump up to the point of takeoff. The mass of the jumper in this case was **63 kg**.

Standing Long Jump Forces:
Jumper Mass = 63 kg

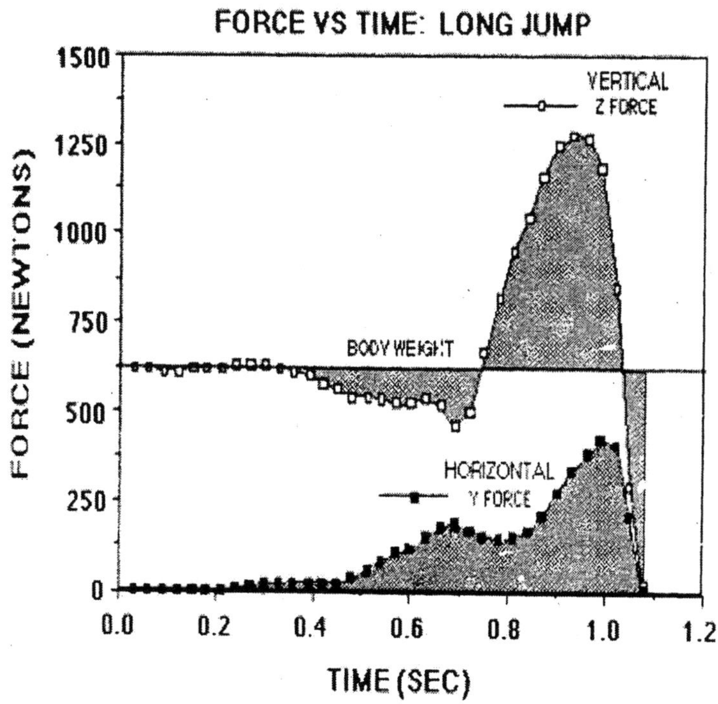

- **Summary Report**

Based on your data analysis and results, briefly summarize the procedures used to determine impulse of ground reaction force. In addition, discuss the meaning of impulse and how it relates to movement that it caused. In your summary and discussion, include responses to the following questions. Limit this writing to one page single spaced. Attach printouts of your *Takeoff and Landing impulse calculations from your own jumps, plus the entire table created for the Standing Long Jump* to the written paper and returns these to your lab instructor at the beginning of the next lab meeting.

Linear Kinematic Analysis

- The purpose of this lab is to provide you with an experience in analyzing video taken with a high speed camera. High speed filming is used for many different reasons in biomechanics. It can be used to measure the release velocity during a baseball pitch, duration of ball-foot contact during a kick or a sprinter's acceleration coming out of the blocks. In today's lab, you will track motion during a standing long jump. Horizontal and vertical positions of the body center of mass will be determined as a function of time.

In the process of making a film or video picture, the image entering the camera's lens is reduced to a fraction of its original size. In viewing the film or video, the images are projected on a screen, viewed on a computer monitor or printed to paper. The images may be smaller or larger than real life size. Because the images are seldom used at real life size, any distance measured on the image must be multiplied by a constant conversion factor to expand it to its real life value.

The standard procedure for determining the conversion factor is to place a meter stick in the camera's field of view during the filming. Knowing the calibration stick's real length and its length when projected, a constant conversion factor can be calculated with the following formula:

$$\text{Conversion Factor (CF)} = \frac{\text{(Real Length of Calibration Stick)}}{\text{(Projected Length of Calibration Stick)}}$$

For example, if a 1 meter calibration stick was placed in the field of view during filming of a runner and then measured as 8 millimeters in the image that was projected from the film, the conversion factor would be:

$$CF = \frac{1\ m}{8\ mm} = 0.125\ m/mm$$

The CF is used to convert distances measured in millimeters on the projected image to real life distance in meters. For instance, if a runner moved 64 mm from beginning to end of a cycle of pictures, the real life displacement would be obtained by:

$$\frac{64\ mm}{1} \times \frac{0.125\ m}{1\ mm} = 8.00\ m$$

Notice that the units cancel to yield a displacement in meters.

It is often necessary to be able to determine time between special events when analyzing high speed film or video. For example, if average running velocity is to be calculated from film images, time is in the denominator of the velocity equation ($V = d/t$). Measuring the time can be accomplished by knowing the number of frames of film between two points of interest and the time per frame.

High speed film cameras usually have adjustable frame rates which are frequently set to shoot between 50 and 200 frames each second (f/s). Video recording is less adjustable. Images can usually be analyzed at 60 or 30 f/s.

The time for one frame of film or video can be calculated from the camera speed setting. For example, if a camera speed of 100 f/s is used, the time per frame is:

$$t = \frac{1}{\text{camera speed}} = \frac{1}{100\ f/s}$$

$$= 0.01 \text{ seconds per frame}$$

This time constant (0.01 seconds per frame) can then be used to calculate time between events. For example, if the above runner (filmed at 100 f/s) took 200 consecutive frames to displace the 8 meters, then the elapsed time would be calculated in the following manner:

Elapsed time =

$$\left(\frac{0.01\ s}{\text{frame}}\right) \times (200 \text{ frames}) = 2.00\ s$$

From the displacement and the elapsed time, the runner's average velocity can be calculated:

$$V = \frac{d}{t} = \frac{8.00\ m}{2.00\ s} = 4.00\ m/s$$

- **Analysis of the Jump**

Enter the horizontal and vertical coordinates for each jump picture into a spreadsheet which will be used for the subsequent analysis.

An unusual characteristic of computer image coordinates that you have recorded is that the vertical coordinate increases as one goes down the image. This is opposite from the "normal" rectangular coordinate system used in mechanics where up is taken as positive. We can easily convert the vertical data to a conventional system by writing a formula in the next column of the spreadsheet. The images you have analyzed had 240 pixels vertically. To set the origin at the bottom left corner as is typical; simply subtract the measured vertical coordinate from 240: (240 - Vert Coord).

Next in the analysis is to convert to real life dimensions in both horizontal and vertical directions. Use the conversion information described above (1 m = 110 pixels) to determine the conversion factor. Then write a formula in the spreadsheet for new columns of real life horizontal and vertical positions (X and Y).

Then, calculate the horizontal and vertical velocity across time using the first central difference formula in the next columns of the spreadsheet.

Finally, to display your results, create graphs of position vs time and velocity vs time for the jump. On each graph include both horizontal and vertical components.

Summary Report

Based on your measured position data and calculations, briefly summarize the methodology and results of this experiment. Discuss how the method might be used for more general analysis of human motion. Include responses to the following questions in your discussion. Limit this writing to one page single spaced. Attach printouts of your graphs and spreadsheet to the written paper and return these to your lab instructor at the beginning of the next lab meeting.

Running Kinematics Lab Write-up Example

There are two factors that determine how fast a person runs: cycle length (CL) and cycle rate (CR). By looking at the horizontal displacement of a person, running speed can be computed by multiplying cycle length by cycle rate. This lab looks at how these two factors affect one's running speed.

Methods

Data were collected in two parts. First, personal data were obtained by measuring CL with a measuring tape. CR was measured indirectly by timing cycles with a stopwatch, then taking the inverse of cycle time (CT). Both of these measures were calculated by taking the average of two cycles to reduce measurement error.

The second set of data were collected from a video file filmed at 15 Hz. CR was found by counting the number of frames involved in one cycle. Treadmill speed was measured before filming and was recorded with each video file. CL was calculated by manipulating the equation Speed=CL*CR.

The measurements were taken to a spreadsheet to be analyzed and graphed.

Analysis

See the attached data table and graphical illustrations of how CL and CR changed with running speed. Generally, CL and CR both increase with speed. However, it is apparent from the data that CR increases much less that CL.

The personal data showed a much greater range of speed. Both sets of data showed CL and CR increasing with CL increasing much more rapidly. The video data showed this with CR only increasing from 1.43Hz to 1.67Hz while CL went from 1.74m to 2.70m. In the personal data, the CR had a low of 1.23 Hz and a high of 1.38 Hz. However, the CL nearly doubled.

The video data probably had a smaller range of error. Error in the video collection came from the low sampling rate. In the measurement of 3 and 3.5 m/s, equal CR's were found because it was impossible to distinguish between the two when counting frames. Error in the personal data came from mistakes in timing, and two measurement markings. While speed probably increased from slow to medium, the cycle rate went down. This may be due to a mistake in starting or stopping the watch.

The magnitude of error in the video file was about 1/30 of a second in timing. In the personal data, timing error was probably around 1/10 of a second and perhaps 0.2 m for the beginning and ending markers.

Kinematics of a Gymnast

- The giant swing is a good example of angular rotation. Your analysis today will be based on figures of a gymnast which were taken from high speed films during a gymnastics competition. A series of images during one revolution of the bar have been combined into a single picture.

- **Methods**

The eleven frames included in the **figure** were uniformly separated in time: **0.15 seconds** between each position. The scaling of the figures can be determined by the meter stick which is included in the diagram.

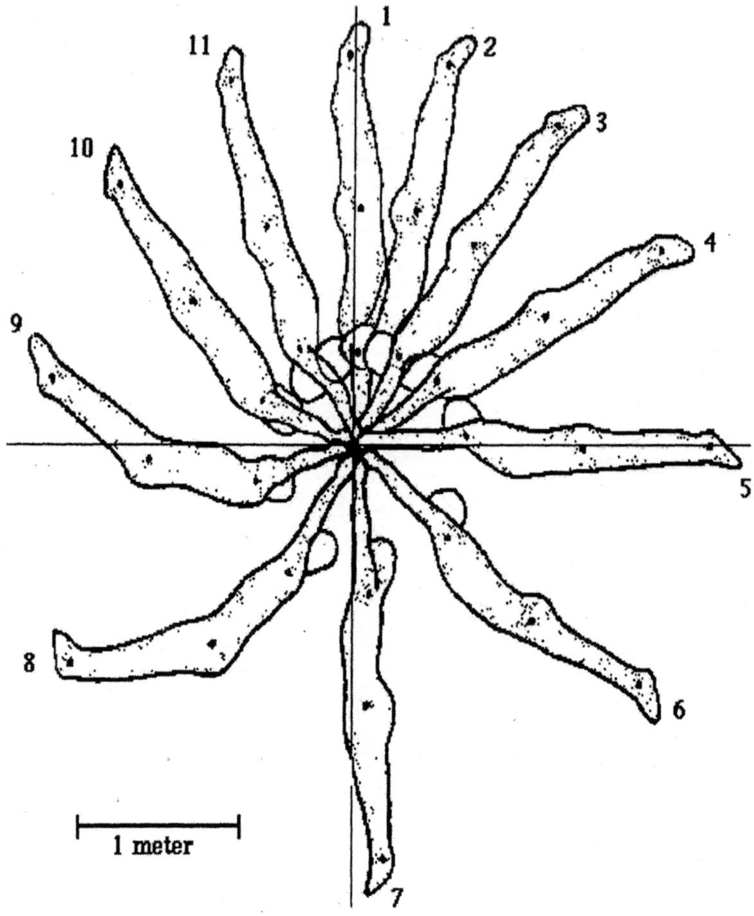

The analysis will involve determination of the gymnast's angular position, angular velocity and linear velocity as a function of time. The reference for the angular measures is the vertical direction. As the gymnast's rotation was in the clockwise direction we will take that to be the positive direction: position 1 being nearly vertical will have an angle of approximately zero. Angles for positions 2, 3, etc. will increase in magnitude till the final position 11 in which the gymnast has nearly rotated through 360 degrees.

To determine the angular position for each of the 11 positions, use the hip marker as an estimation of the center of mass position. Using methods similar to previous labs, determine the coordinates of the hip marker for each position, and also the bar position. From these X and Y coordinates, using trigonometry, determine the angle from vertical for each position. For example at position 3, the hip coordinates are (290, 129) and the bar coordinates are (218, 234). The angle from vertical can be calculated using the arctangent function of (290-218)/(234-129) = 72/105. This corresponds with an angle of 34.4 degrees from vertical.

After determining the angle with the vertical for each frame, you must then determine the angular displacement. In the 1st quadrant (upper right), the displacement is the same as the angle with the vertical. In the 2nd (lower right) and 3rd (lower left) quadrants, the angle with the vertical is formed with the 180° axis. The displacement in the 2nd quadrant is 180° minus the angle with the vertical; in the 3rd quadrant (lower left), the displacement is 180° + the angle. Finally, in the 4th quadrant (upper left), the angle with the vertical is formed with the 360° axis; the displacement is 360° minus the angle. ***Think about this and make sure you understand it!***

Next, determine the radius of the rotation for each frame (distance to the center of mass from the bar). Calculate this distance using pixel coordinates from the screen, then convert to real life dimensions using the meter stick length shown in the figure. For example, at position 3 the gymnast's radius is the distance from the bar to the hip marker. Using the coordinates above in the distance formula, the radius is 127.3 pixels. This converts to approximately 1.29 meters.

Next step in the analysis is to determine average angular and linear velocity during the giant swing. Formulas for calculation of angular and linear velocity during a rotation are:

$$\text{Angular Velocity:} \quad \omega = \frac{\Delta\theta}{\Delta t}$$

$$\text{Linear Velocity:} \quad V = \omega\, r$$

The easiest way to do these computations requires some additions to the spreadsheet. Using **first-central difference formulas,** find the angular velocity for positions 2 through 10. Express these angular velocities in radians per second then calculate the linear velocity for positions 2 through 10.

Finally, illustrate how angular and linear velocity and radius changed throughout the giant swing by graphing the relationships using the spreadsheet data:

1. Angular Velocity versus Angle
2. Linear Velocity versus Angle
3. Radius versus Angle

Graph all the above relationships on the same graph, with angle on the horizontal axis.

- **Analysis**

Summarize your work in this lab with a brief description of methods used for calculating the gymnast's rotational characteristics. Then discuss those characteristics as found in your results. Include responses to the following questions in your discussion. Attach your graphs and spreadsheet to the printout and return these to your lab instructor at the beginning of the next lab meeting.

1. *Where did the greatest angular and linear velocities occur during the giant swing? If they occurred in different frames, explain why*

Angular Kinetics

Human movement is generated through rotations at the joints of the body. The rotations at a joint are controlled by the torques generated by the muscles that act across the joint. In biomechanics, we often combine measurements of body position with simultaneous measurements of ground reaction forces to calculate the resultant torque at a joint during a movement. These resultant torques indicate which muscle groups are most active during different phases of a movement. We can also determine whether the dominant muscle groups are acting to generate power (propulsive phase of movement) or absorb power (braking phase of movement). These provide us insight into the roles of different muscle groups in the control of a movement task.

Remember that the resultant joint torque is the composition of the torques produced by all of the forces acting across a joint. In biomechanics, we compute these resultant joint torques from measured body movements and ground reaction forces using a technique called *inverse dynamics*. In inverse dynamics, we divide the body into rigid segments that are connected at the joints. For each segment, we then use Newtons Laws to derive the equations relating the forces and torques acting on the segment to the motion of the segment:

$$\sum F_x = m\,a_x \qquad \sum F_y = m\,a_y$$

$$\sum T = I\,\alpha$$

It turns out that we can use the measured ground reaction forces and foot movements to solve these equations for the resultant ankle joint force and torque. Then, we can use the computed ankle joint force and torque and the measured leg movements to solve for the resultant knee joint force and torque, and so on up the body.

The sign of the resultant joint torque tells us which muscle group is most active at any given instant during the movement. When looking at a graph of the resultant **joint flexion torque** vs. time, the torque will be **positive** when the **flexors** are generating more torque than the extensors. Conversely, the resultant joint flexion torque will be **negative** when the **extensors** are generating more torque than the flexors. Thus, the flexors are the dominant muscle group during the periods in which the joint flexion torque is positive and the extensors are the dominant muscle group during the periods in which the joint flexion torque is negative.

The dominant muscle group can be used in one of three ways during movement:

1. It can be used to generate power to produce a propulsive (speeding up) action at the joint

2. It can be used to absorb power to produce a braking (slowing down) action at the joint
3. It can be used to hold the joint in a fixed position

We can determine which of these three functions the muscle group is performing by looking at a graph of the power output at the joint vs. time. Remember that, for linear motion, the instantaneous power associated with a force can be computed by multiplying the magnitude of the force by the velocity of the point of application in the direction of the force. Similarly, the instantaneous power output (P) at a joint can by computed by multiplying the resultant joint torque (T) by the angular velocity (ω) of the joint:

$$P = T\omega$$

When the dominant muscle group is **generating** power in a propulsive (speeding up) phase of movement, the joint power output will be **positive**. Conversely, when the dominant muscle group is **absorbing** power in a braking (slowing down) phase of movement, the joint power output will **be negative.** Finally, when the dominant muscle group is holding the joint in a **fixed** position, the joint power output will be **zero.**

Thus, to determine the functions of the flexors and extensors during a movement, we must first determine which muscle group is dominant at each instant. Then, we look at whether power is positive, negative, or zero at each instant.

When the **flexors are dominant** (i.e. flexion torque > 0):

- When the joint **power** is **positive,** the **flexors** are being used to **generate power** and flex the joint faster (propulsion)
- When the joint **power** is **negative,** the **flexors** are being used to **absorb power** and cause the joint to extend more slowly (braking)
- When the joint power is zero, the flexors are being used to hold the joint in a fixed position

When the **extensors are dominant** (i.e. flexion torque < 0):

- When the joint **power** is **positive,** the **extensors** are being used to **generate power** and extend the joint faster (propulsion)

- When the joint **power** is **negative**, the **extensors** are being used to **absorb power** and cause the joint to flex more slowly (braking)
- When the joint power is zero, the extensors are being used to hold the joint in a fixed position

- **Methods**

In this lab, the motion capture system and force plates in the Biomechanics Lab will be used to collect kinematic and ground reaction force data for a countermovement vertical jump by one student. From these data, the software of the motion capture system will compute the knee flexion angle and resultant knee flexion torque for the right knee as a function of time. In your analysis, you will then graph the data, compute the flexion velocity and power output of the knee at each instant, and identify: a) which muscle group, the knee flexors or knee extensors, was most active at each instant and b) whether the muscle group was generating or absorbing power.

In the data collection, a set of 16 reflective markers will be attached to the student at specific anatomical landmarks of the right and left lower limbs. The student will stand quietly on a pair of force plates for 2 s while 8 cameras record the marker positions. Simultaneously, the ground reaction forces beneath each foot will be recorded from the force plates. Following this "static" trial, the student will perform a set of jumping trials. In each trial, the student will begin by standing with one foot on each force plate. When instructed, he/she will execute a countermovement jump. He/she will land with one foot back on each plate and then stand still. Marker position and ground reaction force data will be recorded throughout the jump and landing. Finally, we will measure selected body dimensions of the subject.

Your Lab Instructor will then process the data to do the following:

- Compute the 3-D positions of the markers from the 8 camera images
- Label each of the markers in the resulting 3-D views

- Use the "static" data and body measures to locate the joint center positions and body segment orientations in each trial
- Use these data and the ground reaction forces to compute the torques at each joint by the inverse dynamics technique
- Export the results to an Excel file

You will receive an Excel data file containing the following information for one of the jumping trials:

Column A: Frame #
Column B: Right knee flexion angle (degrees)
Column C: Right knee flexion torque (Nmm)

You will perform the following steps to process the data:

1. For each frame #, compute the corresponding time (in seconds). Because the kinematic data were collected at 120 frames/s, each frame is separated by 1/120 s (= 0.00833 s)
2. Using the central difference method, compute the knee flexion velocity (in deg/s) vs. time. Remember that the formula for the central difference method is:

$$\omega(t) = \frac{\theta(t+\Delta t) - \theta(t-\Delta t)}{2\,\Delta t}$$

Where $\theta(t)$ is the value of the joint angle at time t, $\omega(t)$ is the value of the joint angular velocity at time t, and Δt is the time between frames (You did this before in Lab #5, if you want an example to follow).

3. Convert the knee flexion velocities from deg/s to radians/s.
4. Compute the instantaneous power output at the knee (in milliWatts) vs. time by multiplying the knee flexion torque (in Nmm) by the knee flexion velocity (in radians/s).
5. Using XY (Scatter) plots, make the following 3 graphs for the entire countermovement jump and landing:
   a. Knee flexion angle vs. time
   b. Knee flexion torque vs. time
   c. Knee power output vs. time

6. On your graph of knee flexion torque vs. time, clearly mark the periods of time in which:
   a. The knee flexors were the dominant muscle group
   b. The knee extensors were the dominant muscle group
7. On your graph of knee power output vs. time, clearly mark the periods of time in which:
   a. The knee flexors were being used to generate power
   b. The knee flexors were being used to absorb power
   c. The knee extensors were being used to generate power
   d. The knee extensors were being used to absorb power

In Steps 6 and 7, you must clearly show where each period starts and where it ends.

The RESULTS section of your lab report will consist of the following:

1. A table with the following data in columns:
   - Frame #
   - Time (s)
   - Knee flexion angle (deg)
   - Knee flexion velocity (deg/s)
   - Knee flexion velocity (rad/s)
   - Knee flexion torque (Nmm)
   - Knee power (mW)
2. The three graphs of knee flexion angle, knee flexion torque, and knee power output vs. time. The latter two graphs must include the markings requested in steps 6 and 7 above.

- **Analysis**

In the DISCUSSION section of your report, you will interpret the roles of the knee flexors and extensors in the control of the knee during a countermovement jump and landing. Consider each of the periods you identified in step 7 of the Methods to be a separate phase of the movement. For each phase of the movement from the start of the countermovement until the end of the landing, describe: a) which muscle group is being used, b) what that muscle group is being used to do, and c) what the resulting knee motion is.